EASING LABOR PAIN

EASING
LABOR
PAIN

---

*The Complete Guide
to a More Comfortable and
Rewarding Birth*

ADRIENNE B. LIEBERMAN
Foreword by Penny Simkin

THE HARVARD COMMON PRESS
Harvard and Boston, Massachusetts

To my husband, Syd, in love and appreciation for gifts too numerous to mention, and to Sarah and Zachary, whose births were wonderful despite the pain and who add an irreplaceable zest to my life.

ॐ

16 circ 12/18/98 - 8/99

The Harvard Common Press
535 Albany Street
Boston, Massachusetts 02118

First edition published in 1987 by Doubleday and Company, Garden City, New York.

This revised edition published in 1992 by The Harvard Common Press.

Printed in the United States of America.

Library of Congress Cataloging-in-Publication Data

Lieberman, Adrienne B.
    Easing Labor Pain : the complete guide to a more comfortable and rewarding birth / by Adrienne B. Lieberman ; foreword by Penny Simkin. — Rev. ed.
        p.   cm.
    Includes bibliographical references and index.
    ISBN 1-55832-044-X : $19.95 —
    ISBN 1-55832-043-1 : $12.95
    1. Natural childbirth.   2. Therapeutics, Physiological.
I. Title.
RG661.L54 1992
618.4'5—dc20   92-382

Illustrations by Jean K. Stephens, © Childbirth Graphics, Rochester, New York
Cover design by Joyce C. Weston

10   9   8   7   6   5   4   3   2   1

CONTENTS

ACKNOWLEDGMENTS

Thanks to my childbirth students, past and present, whose narratives and birth questionnaires enliven the facts of this book. I also appreciate the cooperation of the parents whom I interviewed in person or over the phone.

Many professionals speak on the following pages. They graciously took time out of their busy schedules to share expertise in acupuncture, acupressure, biofeedback, massage, hypnosis, therapeutic touch, and transcutaneous electrical nerve stimulation—subjects all previously completely exotic to me. Thanks, also, to the professionals who enlightened me on more familiar subjects.

Penny Simkin, physical therapist, author, and childbirth educator, and Suzanna May Hilbers, physical therapist and former national teacher trainer for ASPO/Lamaze, were kind enough to review the entire manuscript of the first edition. Their comments and suggestions proved tremendously helpful. Special thanks to Penny Simkin for writing such a generous foreword to the revised edition.

The revised edition of *Easing Labor Pain* finally found its true home at The Harvard Common Press. I'm grateful to Lynn Moen of Birth and Life Bookstore in Seattle, who initially suggested The Harvard Common Press, and to my literary agent, Jane Jordan Browne, who oversaw the move. I have thoroughly enjoyed working with editors Dan Rosenberg and Linda Ziedrich, publisher Bruce Shaw, and marketing director Susan Willis—all of whom were eminently available, knowledgeable, and enthusiastic about my book.

FOREWORD

Before the first edition of *Easing Labor Pain* was published, Adrienne Lieberman approached me at a convention, introduced herself, and asked me to read the manuscript for her book. I was slightly jolted when she told me the title—*Easing Labor Pain*—because I was planning to write a book on the same subject. I took the manuscript home, and, after convincing myself that there would be room on the market for two books on childbirth pain, I read Adrienne's manuscript. I loved it. It was what I had wanted to write, only much better.

So, in the course of one day, I gave up my plans to write a book. I contacted Adrienne immediately and enthusiastically praised her extensive understanding of the subject, her marvelous writing style, and her fair-minded approach.

Now, for this updated second edition, she has asked me to write a foreword. I am honored, and it should be easy to write a foreword for a book that I admire as much as I do this one. Yet I have wrestled with it. It has not been easy at all, because the whole subject of childbirth pain is so complex. There are many facets to it, and there is no single way to manage this unique pain. My public, professional childbirth educator self tries to be objective and informative, to give fair and complete information to assist prospective parents in making an informed (and therefore correct) decision.

My other self, the experienced mother and labor support person, who has both felt childbirth pain and has helped hundreds of women cope with it, wants to urge you to prepare for and participate in this challenging life transition. Despite the pain and hard work there is much to be gained from experiencing labor and birth fully. The intangible rewards—closeness with those who help you, intense joy, a sense of accomplishment, and enhanced self-esteem—are felt to a great degree when you work to have your baby.

Easing Labor Pain is full of tried-and-true ways to develop resources both within and outside yourself, all designed to keep the pain of labor within manageable limits. Learn about them, and use them; they will either get you all the way through or far into your labor. Then, if necessary (as with a long or complicated labor), turn to pain medications and other medical interventions for added help. For many women, this approach to birth brings them more than a baby; it also brings the satisfaction of great accomplishment and a sense of fulfillment that are never forgotten.

Happy Birth Day.

Penny Simkin

Introduction to the Revised Edition

You're going to have a baby. You probably don't know your baby's sex. You certainly don't know your baby's weight, hair color, or personality. There's one thing you can count on, though. Having your baby is likely to be painful.

Your best friend told you the pain was excruciating. "Agony," she said, "until I got my epidural block." Your older sister told you it felt like mild cramping, then medium cramping, then *major* cramping—"like being squeezed in a vise grip"—and she even took Lamaze classes. Your mother didn't tell you anything because she didn't want to terrify you. But Carol Burnett revealed that "having a baby is like taking your bottom lip and pulling it over your head."

They're right. Having a baby does hurt. Indeed, that's one thing that hasn't changed at all since this book was first published in 1987.

But lots of other things have changed. Exciting new developments in many aspects of childbearing rendered large parts of several chapters obsolete and dictated the need for a revision of the entire book. In the past five years, for example, we have seen the increased popularity of underwater birth, exercise during pregnancy, single-room maternity care, epidural blocks, and certified nurse-midwives. Traditional delivery rooms and paracervical blocks have practically disappeared.

In addition, as the nation's cesarean rate continued to rise, we applauded as the American College of Obstetricians and Gynecologists revised long-held views on vaginal birth after cesarean and on electronic fetal monitoring. New research vindicated people who recommended female labor support and called into serious question such obstetrical interventions as IVs and episiotomies. In 1989 the American Academy of Pediatrics took a new look at circumcision, cautiously revising its earlier negative stance.

For all these reasons I embraced the opportunity to usher *Easing Labor Pain* into the 1990s. With the addition of well over 100 new references, some chapters changed a lot—the chapters on obstetric interventions and medication, for example—and some changed a little—the chapter on the baby, for example. A few chapters—such as the chapter on relaxation—hardly changed at all. But throughout I have maintained the same purpose I began with in 1987: to help women deal realistically with their fears of labor pain.

Having a baby may be quite manageable or it may be one of the most painful experiences of your life. There are as many different labors as there are women having children. But whether you have twins, breech birth, "gentle" birth, or a cesarean section, you'll need to cope with pain. It's undoubtedly scary, but you have plenty of company.

All ages and cultures have dealt with labor pain. It's a popular myth that ancient or primitive women did not find birth painful and frightening. Even the stoic Greeks chewed willow bark—the predecessor to aspirin—to ease childbirth pain.

In pre-Victorian England, labor pain was considered the lot of womankind. Suffering through birth was the moral thing to do. At least it was until Queen Victoria got those famous whiffs of chloroform for the birth of her eighth child, in 1853.

In the twentieth century in this country, a generation of women demanded and received a medication referred to as "Twilight Sleep," which induced anesthesia *and* amnesia, the better to obliterate both labor pain and its memory. The next generation sought out natural childbirth, a variety of psychological and physical techniques to replace drugs and allow active participation. Birth still hurt, but with preparation and partnership, it became an experience a woman could remember with pride.

Today's expectant parents are offered the very latest in medical technology, an epidural block. The epidural is a medication which relieves labor pain even as it allows awareness and a limited participation in birth.

For some women, this may be an ideal solution, but the situation is actually more complicated than it appears. Unmedicated labor *is* more painful, but completely taking away a woman's birth pain may significantly reduce her pleasure and sense of accomplishment too.

The conflict over how much labor a woman should feel is just one disagreement over the treatment of childbirth pain. Other disputes center over which type of childbirth preparation (if any) is most effective for women, and over whether medication is safe or hazardous to use during labor.

Books that advocate a particular approach usually stress that their method is all a woman needs to know. They give a recipe for a successful birth. But many possible paths lead to the goal of an easier birth. Because each woman benefits from a different approach or combination of approaches, this book doesn't advocate any one form of help to the exclusion of another, nor does it have a strong pro- or anti-medication ax to grind.

Instead, the book explores an eclectic assortment of practical pain-control methods, drawn both from traditional birth sources, and from less traditional areas as well—biofeedback, acupressure, and hypnosis, to name just a few. And for the woman who finds medication necessary or desirable during her labor, this book offers the most balanced and comprehensive discussion of labor medications available to date.

Readers will learn exactly how birth feels to different women, discovering where it hurts, when it hurts, and just what it is that causes the pain of birth. You will find out how the various childbirth education systems, medications, and nonchemical methods actually work, not only to alleviate your labor pain, but to heighten and improve your birth experience at the same time. After becoming acquainted with pain relievers from acupressure to Zen music, you will be uniquely equipped to fashion the most comfortable and satisfying birth possible, both for yourself and for your new baby.

A note on gender: Because of the lack of a suitable, non-sexist pronoun to refer to a baby whose sex is unknown, I have chosen to follow standard English usage and refer to the baby as "him." My apologies to the parents of "hers."

1
Labor Pain

"It was uncomfortable but not painful," said Alice, remembering her nine-hour labor. "I woke up at around 7 A.M. with a tiny backache. My contractions started in the back and went around to the front. They were about ten minutes apart and didn't hurt at all. They kept coming closer until they were five minutes apart. I didn't want to go to the hospital since I was in no pain. By 2 P.M. contractions were four minutes apart and a little uncomfortable. We drove to the hospital where Bill dropped me off at the front door to wait while he parked the car. I chitchatted with the doorman, who asked me if I was there to visit someone. I told him I was there to check and see if we were going to have a baby. He just laughed.

"While I was being examined, the nurse too seemed to wonder what I was doing there. I was sure I couldn't possibly be in labor, but when the resident said I was eight centimeters dilated and almost ready to start pushing, I was the one who started to laugh. After the doctor broke my water, my contractions became very strong and there wasn't any time between them. It didn't really hurt, I just felt like pushing. I pushed for about half an hour and then Alex was born. They gave him to me and I held him. He was so beautiful. To me, having a baby was nothing but pleasure."

But to Sandra, looking back four weeks after the birth of her first child, labor was a "nightmare of pain. Still," she says, "we are so happy with Jessica, I would really do the whole thing again. Now I couldn't say that right after the birth because I hadn't repressed how horrible it was as well as I have now. I can't remember the pain now, but for a week after that labor I could feel this awful sensation in my lower back just where I'd felt the baby's head, or the contractions getting to me for more than 18 hours.

"We had many hours of back labor with repeated attempts by the obstetrician to turn the baby's head to face down. I couldn't endure the pain—maybe someone else could have taken it, but I doubt it. After I received epidural anesthesia, the relief from pain was incredible, like night and day.

"I completed dilating and pushed the baby down over the next twelve hours. She was delivered, without a mark of any kind, with three pushes and outlet forceps. We had a wonderful, joyous, tearful meeting with our new baby, who nursed well in the recovery room. It was the happiest time in our lives. So all's well that ends well, but the labor experience was hellish until I got the epidural."

Between the extremes of Alice's "discomfort but no pain" and Sandra's "nightmare of pain" lie the experiences of most women giving birth. Like Alice, some women experience an easy labor that progresses well with tolerable pain. Others, like Sandra, have a hopeful attitude and a positive approach, but must nevertheless endure a labor that is intensely painful.

Fair or not, labor's really a poker hand. It sure helps to know how to play a good game, and that's what most of this book is about. But despite all your best efforts, what you are dealt in your hand will depend largely on the luck of the draw. One of the best things to remember is that the type of labor you "draw" is not your fault. You just have to do the best you can under the circumstances.

Because it's impossible to know in advance what kind of labor you'll have, you should learn a variety of techniques to help you deal with the many possible variations. In chapters 3 through 18, we'll explore the myriad ways you can help yourself cope with labor pain.

But first you need to know exactly what happens in the course of labor. In this chapter you'll learn what labor is and how it feels; why, where, and when it hurts; why some labors hurt more than others; how labor pain is similar to the pain of a stressful athletic event; and how your body adapts to this difficult experience with a surge of hormones that replace pain with pleasure and perhaps even lead to mother love.

What Happens During Labor

The uterus, where your baby lives and grows for nine months, is a hollow bag of muscles. Labor progresses through a series of contractions (shortenings) of the uterine muscle. These contractions progressively open the cervix (the necklike lower portion of the uterus) until the baby's presenting part (96 percent of the time the baby's head) is in position to be pushed down the vagina or birth canal.

Although you may not notice it, your uterus contracts on a fairly regular basis throughout your pregnancy. You can learn to feel these contractions by placing your hands on the four quadrants of your pregnant belly while sitting or lying down. It feels soft, doesn't it? Now, change your position and feel your abdomen again. It will feel relatively firm all over if your uterus goes into a contraction. Changes of position usually trigger uterine contractions, and they're a perfectly healthy and normal event during pregnancy.

The contractions which lead to the birth of your baby feel both similar to and different from these pregnancy contractions (termed *Braxton-Hicks contractions*). You'll feel your belly tightening and becoming hard, but you'll probably have an even stronger sensation right down inside your pelvis—perhaps in the groin or the low back—because you will also be feeling your cervix thinning out and opening up.

Picture what happens during labor: The uterus must change from the shape of an upside-down gallon wine bottle with a long, closed neck into the shape of a wide-mouthed, open mayonnaise jar. The cervix is first drawn up, or *effaced,* into the body of the uterus, and then the mouth portion is opened, or *dilated,* with the succeeding contractions.

Perhaps a softer analogy would be more apt. The baby, head down, is navigating his way through a tight turtleneck sweater. At first, the neck of the sweater is pulled flat over his head (that's the effacement or thinning-out part) and then the neck opens so that the baby's head can ease through. Because a newborn's head is flexible—the skull bones have not yet fused together—the baby can fit through the cervix when it is dilated to about ten centimeters. (That's about four inches, or the diameter of an average grapefruit.)

The action begins at the top of the uterus, which is called the *fundus.* The long muscles running down the length of the uterus shorten during a contraction, and this shortening pulls at the circular muscles around the cervix. These cervical muscles relax and are drawn back. Luckily, when the uterus stops contracting—and it relaxes fully after each contraction—the long muscles don't revert to their original length, so the space inside the uterus gradually decreases throughout labor, pushing the baby out.

The uterus is a smooth-muscled organ, which means it works on automatic pilot. Of course, you probably know that all sorts of supposedly automatic processes such as heart rate, blood pressure, and yes, even uterine contractions, can be affected by your emotions. We will talk more about that later. For now, let's just say that the best thing you can do to help labor progress in the dilating stage is to "let it happen."

This situation changes dramatically in the next stage of labor, called the second or pushing stage. During the second stage, your uterus continues to contract. Since the cervix is completely opened, there's nothing holding your baby back. At this point, you can add your own efforts to those of the uterus, giving your baby an extra added push to the outside world.

After birth, your uterus continues to contract. The third stage of labor is completed when the placenta or afterbirth is born.

A first-time mother can expect her labor to last an average of about 12 to 18 hours, while an experienced mother can look forward to a shorter labor, perhaps four to eight hours on the average. Averages or textbook labors don't signify much, though, unless you are the rare woman who experiences one. Instead, think in terms of a range of possibilities—your labor can be short, medium, or long and still be absolutely normal, even if it isn't average.

It's especially common to have a very long beginning stage, particularly if this is your first baby. Because labor contractions tend to get longer, stronger, and closer together as you go along, don't fear that a lengthy early stage condemns you to an endless labor process. As time goes by, the pace will definitely pick up, and you will soon be greeting your new baby.

In early labor, the contractions may be very short, only 30 or 40 seconds long, and as far apart as 20 minutes or so. Later, as effacement is completed and dilatation advances, contractions of 60 seconds may come about every three to four minutes. And right before full dilatation, the contractions of the first stage may last as long as 90 seconds, with perhaps only 30 seconds of rest between them. During the pushing stage, the contractions will probably be a little further apart, say about every three to five minutes, and each will last around 60 seconds.

What Does Labor Feel Like?

From the intense, cramping pull or squeeze of the dilating contractions to the profound stretching sensation as the baby's head moves down the birth canal, labor is characterized by powerful feelings. Some women describe the dilating contractions in terms of a more familiar sensation—a cramp, like a menstrual cramp; a charley horse; a gas pain; or a feeling of rectal pressure. One mother says her contractions were like "strong gas pains, tremendous pressure around the pubic area." Another describes labor as "huge waves, like diarrhea cramps, one after the other." Still another says, "My labor felt like extraordinarily severe menstrual cramps with a lot of pressure on the rectum, like constant pressure to have a bowel movement."

Confronting the intensity of pain *before* you give birth may motivate you to learn ways of dealing with it more adequately when you're actually in labor. In fact, a study published recently in *Birth* suggests that women with higher levels of fear before their first childbirth class actually reported *less* anxiety during labor and delivery. The authors concluded that these women probably had dealt with their concerns before they went into labor.

In chapter 13 you'll learn how to put your own images of labor to work for you. One woman, for example, coped with the pain by envisioning the purpose of each contraction: "I visualized my uterus rising up and pulling back, opening the cervix more and more with each contraction."

Why Is Labor Painful?

Now, painless labor is possible—Alice, who opened this chapter, certainly experienced one—but it's quite rare and should always be considered an unexpected bonus.

Labor is usually painful for several very good reasons. For one, the cervix, completely insensitive to burning and cauterization, is nevertheless extremely sensitive to pressure and stretching—precisely what it undergoes during labor. Most women feel contractions as cramping sensations in the groin or back, though some experience more pain in their sides or thighs. As the contractions get longer, stronger, and closer together over the course of labor, they will be perceived as more or less painful by different women.

In addition, the uterine muscle—at term, the largest and strongest muscle in your body—may have to work at alternately contracting and relaxing for hour after hour. That can lead to a tired, achy feeling, just the way the voluntary muscles in your arms and legs might feel exhausted and sore after a difficult workout. The normal decrease in oxygen flow to the uterus as it contracts can add to that achy feeling.

During labor a lot of pressure may be exerted on the fallopian tubes, ovaries, and ligaments. The baby's presenting part (usually the head) presses firmly against your bladder and bowel as he descends through your pelvis. This can lead to great pain, particularly if you don't empty your bladder frequently. About once an hour is a good rule to remember.

The rectum usually empties itself ("nature's diarrhea") in early labor. If it doesn't, you may choose an enema to give your baby more room (see chapter 17). Whether your rectum is empty or not, the pressure of the baby's head on surrounding nerves will be surprising. This feels as though you are going to have a bowel movement *right now*. To some women, that feeling of rectal pressure is extremely painful.

When you are in the pushing or second stage of labor, you will probably feel an extraordinary sensation of stretching in your vagina. "I felt," said one mother, "as if I would burst." Birth is a normal function, of course, but it's hardly an everyday feeling.

When the baby's head comes down to the vaginal opening (this may happen on the first push, but more commonly takes a half hour or more with a first baby), you'll feel a sharp, burning sting as the perineum (the area between your vagina and anus) stretches to accommodate your baby's head. In a couple of minutes, the incredible pressure of your baby's head against the blood vessels and nerves will numb your vaginal opening until several minutes after the birth.

How Much Does It Hurt, Where Does It Hurt, and When Does It Hurt?

We're all familiar with the jokes that make light of labor pain: "I'd rather have another baby than have my tooth filled." We've heard the ones that make labor pain sound bad, too, the ones that celebrate women's strength in getting through it: "If men were the ones who had to have the babies, the population would die out."

How much does it *really* hurt to have a baby?

Dr. Ronald Melzack, professor of psychology at McGill University and a noted pain researcher, helped develop the McGill Pain Questionnaire to answer just such questions. The McGill Pain Questionnaire characterizes different types of pain in terms of their distinctive attributes (like throbbing, burning, rhythmic, pounding, etc.) and also allows a rating of the intensity of any pain on a scale from "none" to "excruciating."

According to Melzack, "Labor is . . . among the most severe pains that have been recorded with the McGill Pain Questionnaire." But while the average labor was indeed rated as very painful, women's scores ranged widely. A few mothers reported easy, almost pain-free labors while others experienced extremely difficult ones.

Whether or not a woman had had a baby before seemed to make a big difference. In an early study, Melzack and his associates queried 141 women, 54 of whom had had a previous baby and 87 first-time mothers. One in four of the first-time mothers rated labor as horrible or excruciating, while only one in 11 of the experienced mothers rated their labors this harshly. The proportions were reversed at the bottom end of the range, with only one in 11 first-time mothers but one in four experienced mothers rating their labors as mild.

Here are the words a significant proportion of the women in this study used to characterize their labors: "sharp," "cramping," "intense," "tiring," "aching," "tight," "throbbing," and "stabbing."

Higher age and socioeconomic status both predicted lower pain scores. Practicing prepared childbirth techniques also seemed to reduce labor pain, a finding other researchers have noted as well (see chapter 3).

Later Dr. Melzack studied 240 women to determine just what accounted for the intensity of their labor pain. Again, he found that first-time mothers experienced more pain. So did mothers who were younger, heavier, or carrying bigger babies, those who had not prepared for birth, and women who reported a history of menstrual difficulties.

Three surprising findings emerged from Melzack's second study:

1. Not all women experienced increasing pain throughout labor. Some women reported high levels of pain consistently, while others had relatively low levels throughout labor. Still others showed the "textbook" pattern of increasing pain.

2. Some of the women felt pain all over the abdomen, back, and perineum, while others experienced pain in more discrete areas.

3. Women with short labors did not necessarily report less pain, nor did women with long labors always report greater pain.

The Pattern of Labor Pain.   Many women find that their labor contractions grow in intensity as labor progresses. A recent study in *Pain* suggests that this is probably a typical pattern. As one woman put it, "I kept thinking it can't get worse than this, but it kept getting worse, and worse, and worse." Another mother recalls contractions during early labor "like strong menstrual cramps which I could walk and talk through. They quickly got stronger, unlike anything I've ever felt."

Some women, however, experience very painful contractions from the beginning. One mother says, "My contractions never felt any more intense or difficult to cope with than they did at the very beginning." Other women find their labor developing in a pattern in which a strong contraction follows a weak one: "I know if this one's easy, the next one's going to get me." A few women find labor mild throughout: "I felt very little pressure, only a little around the baby's head."

The Location of Labor Pain.   While most women feel labor primarily in the groin and lower back, individual women report other locations for their labor sensations: "radiating back to front"; "pressure and pulling on the back"; "pain on either side of my pelvis"; "cramping pain at the top of the thighs, rectal pressure"; "pulling in my lower abdomen, back and side pain"; and "pain in my hips, radiating down my legs."

Particularly if a woman experiences labor mostly in her back, she may find that even while the contractions subside, the back pain doesn't: "With the back pain, it was hard to tell when the contractions began and ended."

The Length of Labor.   A long labor may be exhausting and painful, while a short labor may be easy. A short labor will undoubtedly be termed easy by others, who may say, "You must have had an easy time of it, only four hours in labor!" But a long labor doesn't necessarily imply a painful one and a short labor can be a tumultuous, breathtakingly painful experience. One woman who had a long labor says, "People tend to assume my 40-hour labor was a horrendous experience. But we considered our labor easy because I never felt overwhelmed by my contractions." A woman whose cervix dilated from four to ten centimeters in one hour says, "I've never experienced an hour like that in my life—contractions coming one on top of another—I thought I was dying, the pain was so intense."

Sixty-four thousand American women responded to a *Parents* magazine survey on birth in 1982. Eighty-six percent of the respondents had attended classes in prepared childbirth. Even so, fully one-third of these women said that childbirth was one of the most painful experiences they'd ever had. Another 22 percent said birth was "very painful," 32 percent found it "tolerably painful," 10 percent said "more annoying than painful," and 3 percent said it wasn't painful at all.

Still, when asked which aspect of labor surprised them the most, only one out of five women responded "pain." Thirty-six percent cited "exhaustion," and 19 percent mentioned the length of labor. On the positive side, 26 percent of the women were surprised by the "exhilaration" and 10 percent by "how easy it was."

What do these findings imply for you? If you are typical, your labor probably will be painful. But there is no way to predict in advance how much it will hurt. And no matter what you expect, your labor will probably afford you some surprises.

Pushing: Sometimes a Relief.   Women almost always describe the birth of the baby as exhilarating. But, even before the birth, some women think pushing feels wonderful.

> I could push! What incredible relief. At last I could work with the contractions instead of just enduring them. The hard pain of labor disappeared and was replaced by the most intense feeling I've ever had. I felt triumphant. Where I got the strength from after all those hours I'll never know. I was *so* proud.

> Once I was pushing, there was really no pain, only hard work.

> When I bore down, the pain I'd felt previously diminished. The physical force I was using made the contractions almost secondary; it seemed almost as though they didn't exist.

Just as you might expect, however, some women don't find pushing a relief at all:

> I pushed reluctantly. The back pain peaked and pushing only added to my misery.

> Having looked forward to the "relief" of pushing, I was very disappointed. There was no easing of pain.

> I have never felt such pain as during the pushing.

> As the outer skin of the vagina stretched, it stung incredibly.

Mostly, though, women describe not so much pain as the surprise of how powerful the pushing sensations were:

> Delivery contractions were the most overwhelming and largest experience of my life. I thought my eyes would pop out of my head!

I felt how relentless my body was in its work—how it was forcing me to do a job I had too little strength to do.

Those pushes, coming every one to two minutes, were the hardest, most challenging thing I have ever done.

Birth: The Great Reward.   The moment of birth may be painful—the mother of a ten-pound, two-ounce baby remembers "excruciating pain as the baby's head was born." But most mothers report an extraordinary sensation of relief:

I totally felt the baby's body coming out—it was exhilarating, despite the pain. There was a tremendous release of tension and joy as Jay and I realized we had another boy!

The moment of birth was an incredible orgasmic pain-pleasure which jarred my eyes from the mirror.

Afterwards. Most women find that the pain of birth fades quickly from memory after the baby is born:

The moment of birth is indescribable! The feeling of euphoria and the rush of happiness and newfound strength were wonderful. All the work and all the pain were quickly forgotten in the light of the new addition to our family.

How can I describe such a beautiful yet very painful event when all I see and feel now is the beautiful part? The pain felt during labor has all but been forgotten.

The memory of the pain faded much more rapidly than I would have imagined.

The baby was born at 7:30. Immediately, I experienced what I call a natural childbirth high. It was as though the past 23 hours had never occurred. I was elated.

Some Labors Hurt More

We all know that some labors hurt more than others. It's just not always easy to predict which labors will be more painful. For example, while there are some easy short labors, a very short labor may be experienced as extremely painful because the uterus has to do more work in a briefer period. A woman may have the sense of being tossed into a cold swimming pool at the deep end without the benefit of a warm-up period: "I never had mild, menstrual-like cramping. It was intense, doubling-up contractions from the very beginning."

In several research studies, second-time mothers ranked their births as less painful than did first-time mothers. It's perfectly normal for an experienced mother to compare her second birth to her first. Usually, it *is* easier (or, at least, shorter) the second time around:

> This delivery was an exciting experience. In my first birth, I was hysterical and screaming and just wanted it over with. This time, everything seemed more relaxed and enjoyable.

> Compared to my first labor, which took 36 hours, each one of these contractions seemed to make the same progress as two to three hours of work in the last one.

> With my first baby, I had Demerol which put me on another planet. Still, I couldn't concentrate on anything but the pain, and the contractions just hit me. With this labor, I was alert and could anticipate the contractions.

But birth isn't always lovelier the second time around. A survey of 249 second-time mothers published in the *Journal of Obstetric, Gynecologic and Neonatal Nursing* showed that, although the labors were indeed obstetrically "easier" (shorter, less medication, less blood loss, and fewer forceps and cesarean deliveries), second-time mothers reported the same pain levels as first-timers, perhaps because they received "less support" from their husbands. It could be that if you expect your second or subsequent birth to be much easier than your first, you may experience *more* pain and be less prepared to deal with it. Said one mother, "This was longer and more intense than my first child's delivery. What an unpleasant surprise!"

Instead of assuming that you'll have an easier labor for your second baby, prepare for a difficult challenge each time. If your second labor *is* less painful, enjoy it as an unanticipated pleasure.

Some Labors Really Are Harder

Two types of labors are especially likely to be experienced as painful: labor that is induced or augmented with Pitocin (a hormone that stimulates uterine contractions), and back labor.

Induced Labor.   When labor is induced chemically, women tend to describe the contractions as more difficult than those which occur in a normally progressing labor:

> During my induced labor, we had a terrible time riding each contraction. There was no rhythm to it. We were frustrated and disappointed in ourselves.

There was no time to rest and regroup between the contractions.

The induced contractions started out very strong instead of having a gradual rise to a peak in the middle. It was nearly impossible for me to work with the contractions.

The induced contractions shot through me like a knife.

Experimental research shows that it is harder to cope with pain that comes on very quickly. In *The Challenge of Pain,* Ronald Melzack and Patrick D. Wall write, "Sharp pains that rise rapidly to a peak are especially difficult to control by psychological procedures, while steady or slowly rising pains are easier to control by distraction, relaxation, and other coping strategies."

Even though induced labors end sooner than natural ones, women who are induced use more analgesia and anesthesia for their labors. In a study of 2,182 births, 24 percent of which were induced, researcher Ann Cartwright found that most of the women whose labors were induced preferred not to repeat the experience. This provided a stark contrast to the rest of the women, of whom a majority opted to repeat the type of birth they had experienced. For example, 91 percent of the women having home delivery, 83 percent of all women having their babies in the hospital, and 63 percent of the women having an epidural wanted to give birth this way again, but only 17 percent of the women who were induced said they would want to be induced for a subsequent delivery. In chapter 17, we'll explore several alternatives to induction.

Back Labor.   Most babies begin labor in the head-down position, their faces turned toward the left or right side of your back. In the course of labor, your baby will normally turn to face directly toward your back. This is called an *anterior position*, referring to the relation of the baby's presenting part to a quadrant of your pelvis. Thus, L.O.A., the commonest position, means your baby's skull (occiput, O) is against the left (L) front (anterior, A) quarter of your pelvis.

In general, a posterior position in which the baby's occiput presses against your back leads to a labor in which you feel extreme back pain, hence the term "back labor." Eventually, all but a very few of these babies will rotate to the anterior position before birth—like a key turning to fit a lock. But a few posterior babies will fit through the pelvis to be born "sunny side up"; some will need to be turned anterior with forceps; and, now and then, a "persistent occiput posterior" will have to be born by cesarean.

The baby who spends labor in a posterior position usually gives his mother a severe backache during and even between contractions because his skull is pushing into her backbone. Now it is certainly possible to have a backache during labor without a baby in the posterior position, and it sometimes happens that a baby in the posterior position will spare his mother a backache, but the two—posterior position and backache—tend to be found together.

Childbirth educators commonly put the incidence of back labor at 25 percent, but a study by Rosemary Cogan found that two-thirds of women experience some back pain during labor. About 40 percent of my students answer "yes" to the question, "Did you experience back labor?", on their birth questionnaires.

A study conducted by Ronald Melzack and David Schaffelberg sheds some light on the inconsistent numbers. The authors suggested that women in labor may actually experience two different kinds of back pain, contraction pain and continuous back pain. While three-quarters of their subjects reported some back pain during labor, one-third of their sample of 46 mothers experienced continuous back pain on top of as well as between the contractions. This lingering back pain, the women reported, hurt much more than the pain of the contractions, leading many of them to describe it as "distressing," "horrible," "excruciating," "unrelenting," and "exhausting." The authors suggest that women who experience continuous back pain may need new strategies to cope, such as TENS (see chapter 7).

It's impossible to predict who will have back labor. Low back pain before or during pregnancy does not seem to foretell back labor. Low back pain during menstruation, however, did seem to correlate with back pain in labor in one recent study.

Chapters 4 through 10 in particular will suggest numerous techniques to alleviate the backache that may occur with your contractions or between them. Most women try a combination of different measures, finding different things effective at different times during labor.

Labor as an Athletic Event

The pain of labor has frequently been likened to the ache and exhaustion of a marathon athletic event. Jacqueline Marcus is an experienced marathon runner as well as the mother of three children. "Every time you run, you think you're never going to do it again," says Marcus, "but when you finish, it's wonderful! You did that incredible thing. When you give birth, the experience of making a new life is a hundred times the experience of running, but there's still that same sense of accomplishment, relief that it's over, and awe. With a marathon, you feel proud that you've taken your body through that run. With birth, not only have you taken your body through it, but you've got something to show for it. They are both such incredible physical and psychological feats. To be at the end of a marathon race—it's ecstasy—and so is birth."

The Wall.   In marathon running (as in childbirth), the runner (mother) becomes tired, discouraged, depleted, and ready to give up at some point. Runners call it "the wall," while childbirth educators call it "transition." In a marathon run, the wall comes about 20 miles into the 26-mile race. According to sports psychologist William P. Morgan, writing in *Psychology Today*, the wall is associated with a decrease in glycogen supplies to the muscles and dehydration. Runners begin to feel queasy, dizzy, and light-headed, and as though they can't go on with the race.

In labor the wall may come between around seven and ten centimeters, when the contractions are usually at their strongest and longest, with virtually no rest periods between them. Most women find this tumultuous time during labor exceedingly difficult to navigate.

Beth Shearer, a noted childbirth educator, has observed many Boston marathons and compares the marathon runner to the woman in transition: "People come up Heartbreak Hill (near the end of the race) looking desolate. They're in agony, in terrible pain; they look ghastly. They get to the top of the hill and of course everyone is cheering them on. No one is saying, 'Oh, you poor dear, don't you want anesthesia?' No one is saying, 'Do you want to drop out?' That's not what they need.

"They need encouragement to help themselves go on," says Shearer. "In the marathon, everyone is saying, 'You can do it, you're doing great, just a little bit farther.' They'll get a drink or hosed down if it's a hot day. They get all kinds of physical and emotional support. Once they've scaled that hill, it's downhill and the end is in sight. They're tired and sore, but the triumph of finishing the race can override that."

Before he began his study of marathon runners, psychologist Morgan assumed that the world-class runners would have exotic, extra-special techniques for dissociating their minds from the pain of the wall. Much to his surprise, he discovered that the very best marathon runners flowed *with* the sensations they were feeling during a race rather than focusing their minds elsewhere.

Just as some women never experience a definite transition in labor, some of the runners Morgan studied suggested that the wall didn't exist: "The wall's a myth," said one. "The key is to read your body, adjust your pace, and avoid getting into trouble."

This sounds very much like the advice Australian childbirth educator Julia Sundin gives her clients: "Laboring women can try to lose a little, a little of our need to control, our need to perform, our need to be perfect. Let your head let go of the reins to allow your body to gallop away into labor."

Training for the Big Event. Like an athlete preparing for the Olympics, you may like to try "visuo-motor behavior rehearsal." This combination of relaxation, imagined practice, and the use of imagery strengthens psychological and motor skills as much as an actual rehearsal. One Olympic fencer describes a technique of tension reduction that he uses between matches. In an article in *Psychology Today*, Paul Pesthy writes, "You must be able to stop thinking of the last match, and clear your head before meeting the next one." During labor, each contraction poses a new challenge. If you can clear your mind and relax your body before each new contraction, you will find labor less painful than the woman who stays tense and fearful because the last contraction hurt so much.

Whether or not labor is painful—and to most women it certainly is—the progression in many births echoes the stages in a marathon swim, as described by swimmer Diana Nyad, in an article on the euphoria of marathon swimming: "Hurt, pain, agony, and pleasure, in that order."

Take each contraction as it comes, but keep an overriding focus on the finish line, the moment of birth. One of my students used a poster of a woman runner with the caption "No pain, No gain" to help her focus. When she delivered her baby she said, "I felt high, on top of the world, as though all the pain had never occurred."

Catecholamines and Endorphins: How Your Body Reacts to Pain

When you are in pain or under stress, your body produces chemicals that can make you feel better—endorphins—as well as chemicals that can make you feel worse—catecholamines. Since the two types of chemicals cancel each other out in your system, you should learn how to keep your circulating levels of catecholamines low and how to stimulate your endorphin production. Here's some basic information about your body's chemical response to the stress of labor.

Catecholamines.   Catecholamines—adrenaline and related hormones—are produced in an inborn reflex called the fight-or-flight response. This response occurs automatically when you perceive danger: your hypothalamus (part of the brain) signals the pituitary gland to secrete ACTH (adrenocorticotropic hormone) to the adrenal glands, which respond by pouring adrenaline into your bloodstream. This causes your blood pressure and heart rate to rise. You breathe faster, your senses become keener, your digestive processes stop, and your voluntary muscles tend to contract. Meanwhile, blood is diverted from "nonessential" organs like your uterus. Your pelvis gets rigid, your genitals grow numb, and your anus tightens. You're ready to "fight or flee."

The fight-or-flight response is a lifesaver if you're faced with a menacing stranger in a dark alley. It's a hindrance during labor, for the following reasons:

- Catecholamines slow down your labor by counteracting the hormone oxytocin, which stimulates uterine contractions. This means your contractions will be weaker and farther apart and your labor will last longer.
- Catecholamines decrease the oxygen supply to your baby because blood flow to your uterus is reduced.
- Noradrenaline (another catecholamine) and ACTH (the precursor for adrenaline) suppress endorphin production, and endorphins are your body's built-in painkillers.

It's possible to learn to recognize the fight-or-flight response and it's also possible to learn to turn it off. Here's how. First you should learn to become aware of how your body customarily responds to stress. You can learn how to turn the fight-or-flight response around, primarily by consciously relaxing your voluntary muscles and slowing down your breathing. Turning off the fight-or-flight response takes knowledge and practice, but chapters 4 through 18 are filled with techniques to help you let your labor happen free from unnecessary tension.

Endorphins.   Endorphins are morphine-like chemicals produced by the pituitary gland that cause pain reduction and a heightened sense of well-being. They were discovered in the mid-1970s in a fascinating medical detective story, the brief outlines of which follow.

In studying drug addiction, scientists learned that the body had specific brain receptors for morphine-like chemicals. Since it seemed unlikely the brain would evolve a receptor for a substance produced outside the body, many scientists joined the search for the body's own homegrown painkiller. The simultaneous discovery of endorphins in Scotland and Sweden in 1975 showed that people do internally produce opiate substances, which fit precisely into the brain receptors.

Since endorphins were discovered, some questions have been answered, though many more have been raised. For example, it's been hypothesized that "placebo responders"—that one-third of the population that seems to get relief from a sugar pill or dummy injection—may simply be especially good at producing endorphins. Endorphins, however, are not the only source of pain relief. They play no role in the comfort brought about by hypnosis, for example, and according to some research, they are by no means the only explanation for the placebo effect.

Here is what *is* known about endorphins and labor:

- Endorphin levels rise throughout labor, suggesting that your body works to prevent you from feeling pain.
- Massage, acupressure, acupuncture, and TENS all stimulate endorphin release.
- Endorphins have been found in the placenta and amniotic fluid, suggesting their role as a natural sedative, allowing the baby, too, to feel less pain during birth.
- Endorphins promote the secretion of prolactin, the "motherliness hormone," which leads to feelings of well-being—perhaps the childbirth "high" described by so many women—and the growth of attachment between you and your baby. In laboratory animals endorphins reduce anxiety and irritability and induce the grooming behavior that signifies a caregiving relationship.
- Like jogging, childbirth releases endorphins and prolactin. Thus, the childbirth high may be similar to that experienced by runners after a long, arduous race, a built-in reward for the completion of a difficult task.

What Is Pain, Anyway?

We've talked a lot about labor pain already, but do we really know what pain is? Of course, we're all familiar with pain—we've suffered from headaches and toothaches, hit our "funny" bones, stubbed our toes—but can we define pain? Traditional definitions of pain rely on the customary association of pain with injury: Pain is the sensation that results from bodily injury. But this definition fails to account for injuries that do not result in pain—the striking sagas of soldiers or athletes persisting despite traumas that would, under ordinary circumstances, be painfully disabling. Neither does it account for the spooky but well-documented phenomenon of "phantom limb pain," pain that persists in the absence of physical trauma.

The fact is that pain is a subjective phenomenon, difficult to define precisely. One thing is known for sure, however: Whether or not a sensation is experienced as painful depends on how it is interpreted by the brain. As pain therapist David Bresler puts it, "The main pain receptor is between your ears, for that really is where pain resides."

"Aha," you might think, "so if I don't *think* labor will be painful, it won't be painful." It's not as easy as that, of course, but the fact that pain must be transmitted to your brain and interpreted by it in order to be experienced as pain generates a host of pain-relieving strategies that we'll explore fully in this book.

How Sensation Is Transmitted and Perceived as Pain.   Pain may start anywhere in your body as the result of a painful stimulus—extreme heat or cold, pressure, or injury—which excites pain receptors. The pain signal travels as an electrochemical impulse along the length of the affected nerve to the dorsal (back) horn of your spinal cord. This area runs all along your spine, receiving messages from your entire body. From there, the sensation gets relayed to your brain, first to the thalamus where such sensations as cold, pain, and touch are first processed. Your initial reaction is instinctive—pulling your toe away from a sharp object, for example. Next, the cerebral cortex or thinking part of your brain determines the location and intensity of the stimulus and activates your body to respond; you might then yell "Ouch!" and rub your injured toe.

Pain signals are transmitted primarily by small, slow nerve fibers and—to a lesser extent—by large, fast fibers. Generally, the fast mode of pain transmission ensures your immediate reaction to the pain. The slow fibers account for any lingering ache you'll feel on the injured spot.

Short-circuiting the Pain Message.   It sounds so simple. You get hurt and, sooner or later, you feel pain. Luckily, it's not nearly that simple at all. As it turns out, the dorsal horn of the spinal cord, where messages from all over the body converge before ascending to your brain, acts as a kind of off-on switch, allowing some messages to get through and keeping some messages out. That's right, sometimes pain messages can't get through.

This explanation of pain transmission, known as the gate-control theory, was first formulated by Ronald Melzack and Patrick D. Wall in the mid-1960s. According to Melzack and Wall, the pain gate closes because only a limited amount of information can be processed by the nervous system at one time; when the system gets overloaded, pain signals may be short-circuited. A competing sensation—rubbing the spot that hurts, for example—stimulates large, fast-moving nerve fibers conveying touch and this closes the gate to the small, slow-moving pain messages.

Acupuncture, massage, and TENS probably also halt pain transmission by stimulating the secretion of endorphins, your body's built-in pain relievers.

Psychological factors, too, play a vital role in the control of pain. Attention or nonattention to pain can open or close the gate of pain perception, allowing more or fewer pain messages to get through. Anxiety, relaxation, anticipation, and past experience are all examples of descending messages that can shut or open the way for the pain messages.

What's Your Pain Threshold? Based on past experiences, most people tend to evaluate their ability to withstand pain as high or low. Actually, four different thresholds have been measured in laboratory tests on tolerance for pains like electric shock or ice-water immersion. As you will learn, most of these thresholds are highly variable, which should give you great encouragement even if you're convinced you have a "low" pain threshold.

- *Sensation* threshold is the stimulus value at which a sensation such as tingling or warmth is first felt.
- *Pain-perception* threshold is the stimulus value at which a person reports the stimulus as painful.
- *Pain-tolerance* is the stimulus level at which a person withdraws or asks to have the stimulus stopped.
- *Encouraged-pain-tolerance* is the level at which a subject withdraws or asks to have the stimulus stopped after being encouraged to tolerate higher levels of pain.

People of all cultures seem to share a uniform sensation threshold. In other words, most people start to feel a sensation at the same intensity.

But the level at which people report the stimulus as painful is affected by their current condition. For example, experimental research suggests that pregnant women seem to have increased pain thresholds as labor approaches. Past experience and cultural background may also change the meaning of the situation to make it more or less painful. One study, for example, showed that women who had previously experienced high levels of pain unrelated to childbirth reported less labor pain than other women.

Another recent study compared Dutch and American women giving birth. American women were much more likely to expect labor to be painful and to assume that they would need medication for it. They predicted correctly. Indeed, only one in six American women received no medication compared to almost two-thirds of the Dutch women.

The biggest difference among people, however, isn't in their perception of pain but in their ability and motivation to withstand it. In one experiment, for example, Jewish women increased their level of tolerance *after* they were told that their religious group had a lower pain tolerance than others.

It's well known that a person may have a low tolerance for pain in one situation, but a high tolerance in another. For example, soldiers whose severe wounds would warrant strong painkillers in a civilian population nevertheless denied feeling high levels of pain when they were interviewed away from the battleground. Athletes are often observed to continue playing despite injuries that a non-player probably would find quite painful.

Your pain threshold can also be lowered or raised by the type of attention you focus on a sensation. In one pain experiment, simply reading the word "pain" in the instructions made subjects find a low level of electric shock painful. They didn't report the same level of shock painful when the suggestive word "pain" was left out of the instructions. This, of course, is the reason childbirth teachers refer to "labor contractions" and not to "labor pains."

By the same token, if your anxiety is reduced instead of built up, your pain threshold may be increased. Another pain experiment gave subjects control over the painful stimulus, an electric shock. With a sense of control, subjects found the stimulus less painful, probably because they experienced less anxiety about what would happen to them.

Reducing Labor Pain.   Because pain perception is so malleable, you can reduce the pain you feel during labor in a variety of ways. You may be able to alter the physical sensation itself, say, by changing your own position (see chapter 10). Perhaps you'll choose to intercept the pain message, closing the gate or jamming the transmission of pain by sending competing soothing messages—counterpressure, massage, or TENS are but a few of the means to do this.

You'll probably also use many psychological methods of restructuring the pain messages, like tuning into your body and employing positive imagery to reinterpret painful sensations as "opening" or "the baby descending." You can soothe yourself with attention-focusing devices such as relaxation, slowed breathing, and music; and you can supply yourself with calming sights to look at, and special companions to comfort you. Perhaps you'll choose to concentrate on so-called left-brain (rational) activities—counting to yourself, pacing or patterning your breathing, focusing on a particular picture, or listening to your partner count time on a watch. Practicing lots of strategies and being flexible about changing strategies midstream can help you get through the painful contractions and prevent you from tensing up in anticipation of future pain.

All these techniques represent merely the tip of the iceberg of methods you can use to lessen the pain of birth. Many ways exist to respond to the challenge of bringing a new life into the world, and we'll explore a good number of them in detail. With education, practice, and commitment, you'll be well equipped to help yourself alleviate pain and get the most out of your birth experience.

Something Important to Keep in Mind

If you found yourself tensing up as you read the descriptions of labor pain and the body's reaction to stress, take a calming breath. Labor pain *does* exist for most women, but you can do a lot to make it more tolerable. Under ordinary circumstances, the pain of labor is not the pain of trauma or of bodily injury. It *is* the pain of intense effort, but it usually fades quickly after the effort is spent. Experienced labor and delivery nurse Dinah Hobart puts it this way: "Labor pain is a productive pain, a positive pain. The stronger the pain, the sooner the baby will be born. Your intent with other pain is to take it away, but with labor, you try to work with it more than trying to take it away."

Remember, too, that unlike some kinds of pain, labor pain is usually intermittent, not continuous. Furthermore, it is fairly predictable, it has a definite ending, and, best of all, you get an extraordinary reward at the end. As one new mother says, "At my first glance at her tiny presence, I decided unhesitatingly that every second of the pain had been worth it. I would do it all again for such a beautiful result."

2
The Myth of
the Painless Birth

Despite the fact that labor is painful for most women, a powerful myth of painless childbirth still prevails. Deep in our minds, many of us feel that if we could only prepare better, practice more, give birth in the "right" circumstances, or alter our cultural bias from high tech toward a more "natural" style of childbirth, then labor wouldn't hurt.

The attitude that birth *shouldn't* hurt can still be found in popular books that proclaim, "Pain is neither necessary nor inevitable in a normal labor." Indeed, as women today we have control over so many aspects of our lives it's almost impossible to imagine we shouldn't also be able to overcome labor pain, too.

The myth of painless childbirth actually springs from the original books on prepared childbirth—written by men—and from our wishful image of the woman in an underdeveloped country who squats momentarily in the bush to give birth, then resumes her wholesome outdoor work without missing a beat. The feeling that we too could have painless births if only we, or the system, or our culture were different has promoted widespread feelings of anger, guilt, and inadequacy in many of us. For if labor isn't supposed to hurt and mine does, then either I've done something wrong or my labor must be abnormal.

This chapter examines the myth of the painless birth from its dual origins to its effects on American childbirth today. We'll take a look at how birth really is (or was) in other parts of the world and suggest some important contributions anthropology can make to an improvement of Western-style birth. Finally, we'll explore some ideas about the function of pain in a normal labor in order to question the popular assumption that a painless birth is necessarily a better birth.

Grantly Dick-Read and Fernand Lamaze: Learning to Do Birth "Right"

Childbirth education in America bears the stamp of two European obstetricians, who came independently to radical turning points in their respective careers of delivering babies to routinely anesthetized mothers. Grantly Dick-Read, the British founder of the natural childbirth movement, was converted one rainy night before World War I as he delivered a baby to a poor woman who refused his offer of chloroform with the words, "It didn't hurt. It wasn't meant to, was it, doctor?"

In his 1944 book *Childbirth Without Fear*, Dick-Read said: "For weeks and months afterwards, as I sat with women in labor, women who appeared to be in the terror and agony of childbirth, that sentence came drumming back into my ears—'It wasn't meant to, was it, doctor?'—until finally, even through my orthodox and conservative mind, I began to see light. I began to realize that there was no law in nature and no design that could justify the pain of childbirth."

Dick-Read believed that women's fears of birth—generated by other women, their husbands, the media, religion, and doctors—caused the very tension that made labor so painful. According to this theory, if fear could be eliminated through education, and tension reduced by relaxation training, childbirth could again become the joyous, pleasurable, and painless event Dick-Read assumed primitive women experienced: "Civilization and culture have brought influences to bear upon the minds of women which have introduced . . . fears and anxieties concerning labor. The more cultured the races of the earth have become, so much the more dogmatic have they been in pronouncing birth to be a painful and dangerous ordeal."

Fernand Lamaze was a French obstetrician whose enlightenment came in the Soviet Union in 1951. He had gone there to observe psychoprophylaxis (literally, mind-prevention), Pavlovian conditioning techniques applied to eradicate the pain of labor and eliminate the need for drugs. "I had at the time," said Lamaze, "thirty years of experience as an obstetrician and had never been taught anything like this. I had never seen it; nor had I ever thought it could be possible. My emotional reaction was therefore all the stronger. I made a clean sweep of all preconceived ideas and, now an elderly schoolboy of sixty, I immediately decided to begin studying this new science."

Like Dick-Read, Lamaze felt that labor pain was caused by psychological and social factors. Since the expectation of pain had been conditioned, thought Lamaze, it was not part of the natural experience, and so it could be erased by a process of reconditioning. This reconditioning consisted of rigorous training in relaxation and breathing patterns to substitute a positive response for the traditional pain response.

Psychoprophylactic training required a major effort on the part of the woman, who, according to Lamaze, must be "imbued with the thought that she is essentially responsible for the success or failure of her own childbirth. . . . Her mind, carefully educated, steadfast and alert, will know how to abolish pain."

Both Dick-Read and Lamaze believed that pain in childbirth resulted from faulty education about birth. Through a process of reeducation, a woman following Dick-Read's or Lamaze's approach could therefore expect to give birth without pain. For Lamaze, childbirth education was rational, matter-of-fact: "A woman learns how to give birth in the same way that she learns how to swim, or write or read; and she does so without pain." For Dick-Read, painless birth was mystical, religious, "the natural reward of those who perfect their ultimate purpose in life." But despite their differences in tone, both doctors emphasized that a normal birth should be painless.

The idea that unmedicated birth could be painless was a terribly radical one for the era. Around the same time the Englishman Dick-Read had his initial revelation about painless childbirth, American women were organizing to pressure their doctors into drugging them for painless birth. It seems ironic now, but the very women who founded the Twilight Sleep Association were among the most well-educated and liberated women of the time. Reformers, suffragettes, and advocates for birth control and improved working conditions all joined to promote "twilight sleep" as one more way to liberate women from pain and indignity.

The "painless birth" sought by the Twilight Sleep Association required a hospital setting. When birth in America took place at home, doctors had but a limited arsenal for pain relief; they could give ether, chloroform, or nitrous oxide with oxygen at the very end of labor. Between 1915 and 1948, American mothers moved en masse to hospitals where they received a panoply of new medications for labor and birth: narcotic and nonnarcotic analgesics; barbiturates and other sedatives; hypnotics; tranquilizers; local, regional, and general nerve blocks. Singly or in combination, these medications were given orally, rectally, hypodermically, by inhalation, or by injection from early labor throughout delivery.

After World War II, when Lamaze was learning psychoprophylaxis in Russia, most American women got routine anesthesia for birth. But some women found the side effects of the painkilling drugs more unpleasant than the pain that had preceded them. Doctors, too, began to notice that these drugs affected the newborn baby.

Dick-Read's ideas had begun to filter across the Atlantic even before the American edition of his book was published in 1944. A pilot program at Yale University began to implement natural childbirth in the 1940s. Despite some interest in Dick-Read's ideas, however, American childbirth didn't really change very much until 1959 when Marjorie Karmel's book *Thank You, Dr. Lamaze* came out. Karmel, an American woman, had experienced a painless first birth in France under Dr. Lamaze's care. When she came back to the United States, she wanted to spread the good word. With the establishment of the American Society for Psychoprophylaxis in Obstetrics (ASPO/Lamaze) in 1960, the Lamaze method became the prevalent system of childbirth education in the United States.

Interestingly enough, Dick-Read's and Lamaze's assumption of painless childbirth as the norm never won universal acceptance, even by some of their most avid followers. For example, Frederick Goodrich, an early advocate of Dick-Read's natural childbirth theory, reported in a 1949 paper on the Yale program that only two percent of 400 women deemed their labors painless. Goodrich found that the Dick-Read approach made women's labors less painful and more positive, but he concluded that completely painless childbirth was very unusual. Even the Soviet scientists who originated the psychoprophylactic method—which came to be known as the Lamaze method—soon began to feel that not all the pain in childbirth was learned or conditioned.

Both Dick-Read and Lamaze had similar aims: to give information, to alleviate unnecessary fears of birth, and to substitute relaxation for tension. These aims still form the basis of today's childbirth education programs. But a lingering legacy of distrust continues to surround childbirth education because of its historic association with the idea that childbirth could or should be painless.

Today's well-educated parents, more likely than not to take childbirth education classes, may still be laboring under the delusion that the classes will take all their labor pain away. When this fails to happen, as it usually does, they may blame themselves—"If only I'd practiced more, or breathed correctly, or had my baby at home"—or they may blame their childbirth instructors. In her 1990 book, *I Wish Someone Had Told Me*, Nina Barrett writes, "From my Lamaze classes, I picked up the idea that an earnest and positive approach to childbirth would foster a pleasant experience." She continues, "Natural childbirth advocates deliberately airbrush their language, referring neutrally to 'powerful sensations' and 'hard work.'"

Both Dick-Read and Lamaze thought that even to suggest the possibility of pain would cause the very pain that was suggested. But when the reality of pain is denied, women end up feeling frustrated, angry, and unprepared. As Nina Barrett puts it, "One of my first thoughts after labor was finally over was: 'Why didn't anyone tell me that it *hurts*!'"

As we'll learn in chapter 3, most current childbirth educators face the reality of pain in labor more honestly than they did a few years ago. This openness should help dispel the widespread perception of childbirth education as a whitewash. But there's still the other thread of the painless-birth fantasy to follow: the "noble savage" theory. Many of us believe that "primitive" women gave (or give) birth without pain, and that if we were just more like them, we could do it too.

Somewhere, Somehow, the Women All Give Birth Painlessly . . . or Do They?

In 1975, Suzanne Arms's book *Immaculate Deception* challenged traditional American childbirth practices in a style that combined passionate fervor with carefully marshaled research. Arms castigated obstetricians for a host of practices that lacked scientific justification: induction, episiotomy, anesthesia, and the routine separation of mothers and babies. Her book aptly condemned "an entire system of medical procedures and interferences [that] had been established to treat normal birth as a risky, dangerous, painful, and abnormal process in which pregnant women have no choice, other than to submit graciously."

But Arms was treading on shakier ground when she asserted that "primitive woman did not expect what we call 'pain in childbirth'

. . . . Pain to [primitive woman] was associated with unnatural occurrences such as sickness and injury." Taking a leaf from Grantly Dick-Read, Arms suggested that modern society had made birth complicated and difficult; by contrast, primitive women approached birth "with a matter-of-fact acceptance and without fear or expectation of pain."

It's impossible to subject statements like that to proof, but in every place anthropologists have studied birth, they have found painless birth to be the exception instead of the rule.

Probably because we tend to feel that what is "natural" must be "good"—witness the appearance of organic foods on our supermarket shelves—we assume that birth in nonindustrial societies must be more natural and hence easier, shorter, and less painful than our own. But human childbirth does not occur in a cultural vacuum anywhere on earth. Every society has elaborate rules as to who may come to birth, what should happen, and how the participants must behave. And every culture has evolved techniques to deal with prolonged or painful labors.

What do we know of birth in traditional society? The most thorough account remains Margaret Mead and Niles Newton's 1967 study, in which they reviewed the anthropological literature to date on 222 cultures. In every culture, pregnancy was treated as a special condition. Dietary and sexual restrictions, prescribed rituals, and avoidances prevailed. All cultures placed a particular importance on birth, but some treated it as an illness while others did not. For example, while the Hottentots limited a laboring mother's physical activity, the Tuareg of the Sahara encouraged mothers to walk throughout labor. Some cultures opened childbirth to many participants, while others relegated birth to a secluded place. Far from the mythical image of a solitary woman having her baby unceremoniously and returning to work without ado, most cultures provide at least two or more attendants for birth and conduct birth in a hut that has been specially built for the occasion. The recovery period after traditional birth is often prolonged as well. It's hardly a casual or solitary affair.

Furthermore, "primitive" labor frequently gets a chemical or nutritional boost. Societies have used varied concoctions; the Amhara of Ethiopia, for example, thought mashed linseed would relax the birth tract and lessen pain. More than a few societies employed plants to ease suffering, and while some cultures, including our own, limited eating and drinking during labor, others encouraged a woman to keep up her energy by taking in food and drink.

Perhaps the element that most distinguishes birth in traditional cultures from birth in our own is company. In most societies, familiar helpers—most always women, but often the husband as well—cheer on the laboring woman with their encouragement and solicitude.

Anthropologist Brigitte Jordan describes traditional birth in the Yucatan in her book *Birth in Four Cultures*. Jordan became the confidante of a native midwife. She participated at the childbirths of a number of Mayan women; in her book, she compares these births to births she observed in the United States, Sweden, and Holland.

In the Yucatan, a husband is expected to be present during labor so he can "see how his wife suffers." If her labor is long, an entire entourage of people—mother, mother-in-law, grandmothers, sisters and sisters-in-law, close friends, and neighbors—filter in and out to relieve one another and to lend the woman their emotional and physical support. It's universally accepted that labor often takes a long time, but most of these participants have given birth themselves, so they keep reminding the mother that her own baby will soon be born. Their encouragement even includes scolding if the mother needs it, but the laboring woman always knows that she will never be left alone.

What do the helpers do at a traditional Mayan birth? One in particular sits behind the mother on a hammock, with her arms under the mother's shoulders, supporting the mother's body on her lap. This helper pushes the mother up at the peak of the contraction and supports her when she rests back down. The other helpers rub the mother's abdomen, her back, her lower legs, and her thighs. They also engage in "birth talk," a swell of voices rising in a stream of words whose intensity matches that of the mother's contractions. Jordan writes, "The laboring woman is surrounded by intense urging in the touch, sound, and sight of those close to her."

Birth is painful for Mayan women. But the pain is universally recognized as a normal part of childbearing. A child will be born, it is said in the Yucatan, in "the center of the pain." Pain is seen as the very hallmark of labor progress rather than as a symptom to be treated or an evil to escape.

No known culture, traditional or modern, expects childbirth to be painless. Still, there's a lot to learn from cultures other than our own.

Traditional cultures use nutrition and herbal remedies, massage and manipulation, upright postures and activity, a rich variety of sensory stimuli including music, and, perhaps most important of all, the support of experienced companions to urge the mother on. These and the other methods of relieving pain we'll discuss in the remainder of this book will certainly help you more than the myth of the "painless" primitive childbirth. No "quick fixes" can alleviate the pain of birth, but you can certainly learn how to comfort yourself more efficiently.

Why Is Labor Painful?

As we've seen, declaring that labor won't hurt and constructing theories about why it shouldn't hurt haven't stopped most women from actually feeling labor pain. What isn't well understood is just why birth *does* hurt. While no definitive answers exist, Aidan Macfarlane suggests several interesting possibilities in his book *The Psychology of Childbirth*. For one thing, Macfarlane writes, the vagina and perineum are exquisitely sensitive to pleasurable sensation. Perhaps pain fibers are necessary in these areas to protect them from damage, just as pain sensation in any part of the body serves as an alerting mechanism to keep us from hurting ourselves.

Labor pain can and does function as a useful signal. For example, the pain of uterine contractions usually prompts a woman to get to a safe place before she gives birth. This pain may also induce her to change positions or to ask for a massage.

Lower animals don't suffer as much in giving birth. In more intelligent animals, however, we begin to see both birth pain and the need for extended maternal care of the young after birth. Perhaps labor pain plays a role in increasing motherly feelings, which may be promoted by the endorphins and prolactin mothers produce after birth.

In some experiments animals anesthetized for birth showed altered behavior toward their young, at times rejecting them. Of course, human beings adapt more easily to varied birth practices. But it could be that pain during birth functions somehow to enhance maternal behavior.

At the very least, pain tends to keep a new mother alert. First labors, in particular, usually take a long time, but most new mothers feel wide awake after birth for at least an hour or two. Fortunately, this is a period of extreme alertness for newborns as well, even though babies will be sleepy afterward for the next few days. Perhaps pain and its sudden cessation serve to counteract the natural exhaustion that can follow a stressful undertaking.

Is a Painless Birth
Necessarily the Best Birth?

Considering the variety of medications offered and consumed during a typical Western birth, it seems that many doctors assume a painless birth is the best birth. Mothers may or may not agree. For example, a British study of maternal satisfaction with childbirth investigated

1,000 women who had had vaginal deliveries. In this study, epidural block was deemed the most effective pain reliever, but women who received epidurals expressed more dissatisfaction with their labors than women who labored without anesthesia. As it turned out, women related unhappiness in labor not to pain but rather to forceps delivery and long labor, both of which prevailed in the epidural group.

In fact, birth does not have to be painless to be experienced as exhilarating. Years ago, Deborah Tanzer, a psychologist, studied the effect of Lamaze preparation for birth and published her findings in a book called *Why Natural Childbirth?* Tanzer was particularly interested in whether prepared childbirth students were likely to have a "peak experience," Abraham Maslow's concept of an ecstatic happening. Tanzer's results showed that prepared women were much more likely to have a peak experience at birth; furthermore, it was entirely possible for a woman to experience extremely high levels of pain and yet, at the same time, describe her birth as "rapture." In other words, having a peak, ecstatic birth experience did *not* require feeling no pain.

This will not come as a complete surprise if you consider that pain and pleasure actually form two poles of the same process, sensitivity to feeling. Rather than opposing each other, pain and pleasure stand together as the opposite of a lack of feeling.

Our culture tends to stress an avoidance response to pain, not experiencing and learning from it, but, rather, escaping from it into insensitivity. We assume that what leads to pain must be bad and should be remedied. But the experience of pain may actually help you to feel a deeper pleasure.

Whether or not you choose drug-free childbirth, don't make the mistake of assuming that pain in birth only happens if you are not breathing right or haven't got the correct mental attitude. If you labor under the misconception that you're going to feel nothing stronger than "discomfort," you'll probably be brought up short by the reality of intense pain. On the other hand, if you anticipate pain as a natural part of your birth process, you might actually relish the experience of meeting this difficult challenge head on.

Sometimes a woman learns something surprising about her own ability to handle pain during labor. Before she had her first baby, Nancy Reese was sure natural childbirth was an idea whose time had come—and gone. She says, "I let everyone, including my Lamaze teacher, know I wanted as many drugs as I could get during labor."

As things turned out, Reese got quite a surprise during labor. Over two days, her contractions varied from two to 20 minutes apart, but never became regular enough to send her to the hospital. She stayed home, eating lightly and taking warm baths to stay relaxed. She used her breathing techniques and tried some of the different positions she had learned in class—rocking on hands and knees and squatting with the aid of a kitchen chair. By the time Reese arrived at the hospital, she was almost completely dilated, and it was too late for her to get the drugs she had been so sure she would need.

Looking back on her drug-free birth, Reese observed, "I wouldn't do it any other way. It was absolutely wonderful. As soon as delivery was over, I felt so good. Jonathan was with us in the recovery room, just as alert as he could be."

No matter what type of labor you have, your baby's birth is unlikely to be painless. But with adequate preparation for childbirth— the subject of the next chapter—you can give up the self-indulgent and disappointing fantasy that your labor should be painless and replace it with a more realistic and ultimately more rewarding commitment to working *with* your pain.

3

Childbirth Education:
The More You Know,
the Less It Hurts

The childbirth education movement grew out of two ideas: first, that labor was not intrinsically painful, and second, that with good training any woman could have a painless birth. Now that we know that birth is painful even for prepared women, does that make childbirth education a waste of time? Not if class attendance is any indication. Four out of five first-time expectant mothers attended childbirth classes in 1990.

Doing away with childbirth education because labor is still painful truly would be a case of throwing the baby out with the bathwater. For even if childbirth education can't take away all the pain of birth, it certainly reduces suffering. What's more, widespread education has done much to transform women's experience of birth from a hazy nonevent to a joyous family beginning, an occasion to be remembered with pride.

This chapter will show how childbirth preparation can reduce labor pain and will acquaint you with what goes on in a typical childbirth class. We'll compare classes with different philosophies and you'll learn how to select the best childbirth class and instructor to meet your own needs.

How Does Childbirth Education Reduce Labor Pain?

Research reports from numerous institutions clearly demonstrate that education for childbirth reduces pain for most women. Moreover, compared to unprepared mothers, women who prepare for birth use fewer medications, have a lower rate of forceps deliveries, and express a more positive attitude toward childbirth. Clinical studies of surgical patients show similar results: patients who receive information on what feelings and procedures to expect, and instructions on how to relax, have significantly reduced postoperative pain and use much less medication than unprepared patients.

The evidence remains divided on whether childbirth preparation makes for shorter labors with fewer complications. Some studies say it does. Other researchers contend that findings of shorter labors and fewer complications come from the fact that women who take childbirth preparation classes typically use fewer medications.

What is clear is that prepared women are calmer and more relaxed during labor. They remember labor as a more positive experience than do women who are unprepared. As one woman said, "The things I learned in class didn't take all the pain away, but rather gave me the ability to cope with it. Plus, I didn't create more pain by fighting the process."

The Nuts and Bolts of Childbirth Classes

Regardless of the type of childbirth classes you choose, all preparation for childbirth shares the same three basic components: *education* about birth and hospital procedures; *emotional support* from the group and instructor; and *practical techniques* for coping with birth.

Education in childbirth classes includes charts and discussions of fetal development and the dynamics of labor and delivery. Classes often cover related topics, too, such as nutrition, sexuality during pregnancy and postpartum, pros and cons of hospital procedures and of medications for labor and delivery, characteristics of newborn babies, parent-infant attachment, infant care and feeding, concerns of new parents, and sibling relationships. Most classes include information on cesarean birth. Many incorporate movies, slides, or videotapes.

Emotional support is built into the very design of group classes. Meeting with other people who are going through the same process relieves anxiety as you learn that you're not alone in your feelings and concerns. Your husband or partner also learns effective ways to support you through labor.

Practical techniques to cope with labor include different methods of relaxation, attention focusing, patterned breathing, position changes, comfort techniques, meditation, and imagery.

Classes may begin in the early or middle part of pregnancy or they may be designed specifically to be taken during the last two months. An early class—or ongoing instruction from the middle of pregnancy—can promote good posture and get you started on exercises and relaxation techniques. Other childbirth classes are particularly scheduled for the end of pregnancy to take advantage of your heightened motivation at that time to learn coping strategies for labor and delivery.

If you plan to take classes only at the very end of your pregnancy, don't wait until then to register; in some areas, classes fill up very quickly. You'll want to leave enough time to research what is available in your community and perhaps even to interview or observe several different instructors. Call early, and you may be able to take advantage of "early-bird" classes on nutrition and exercise.

Why Take a Childbirth Class?

Books on childbirth preparation abound, and audiocassettes and videotapes now are widely available (see Resources). If you are highly motivated, you can learn some basic childbirth skills from a book or tape, but try to take a class if you can.

First, you'll get invaluable support from other people who share your concerns about giving birth and becoming parents. You'll also appreciate an experienced instructor who can help you know whether you are, in fact, learning to relax.

Sharron Humenick, associate professor of nursing at the University of Wyoming, says that learning to relax is "one of the few skills couples can't get from a book—only from a teacher." Studying women who had been trained to relax for childbirth, Humenick found that the better they were rated at relaxing, the less pain medication they used in labor. In class, the teacher will train your labor partner to check you for relaxation (see chapter 4).

A study in the *Journal of Obstetric, Gynecologic and Neonatal Nursing* compared class-taught Lamaze students to a group of women who had taught themselves Lamaze. The class-taught women practiced relaxation more frequently before giving birth and they had a higher degree of relaxation in labor than the women who trained themselves.

If your practice time is limited, take heart. It doesn't take a lot of practice in prepared childbirth techniques to reduce labor pain. Practicing relaxation techniques for five to ten minutes a day and patterned breathing for ten to 15 minutes a day, especially if you practice along with a partner, significantly reduces the amount of pain women report during labor. More isn't necessarily better: longer practice times don't reduce pain any further.

Which Childbirth Class Should You Take?

In large metropolitan areas, you may have many types of childbirth-education philosophies and instructors to choose from, while in other areas, your choices will be more limited. For further information on the organizations and childbirth methods described below, see the Resources section at the end of the book. Most childbirth organizations will be glad to give you a list of certified teachers in your area.

You should know that childbirth instructors frequently take an eclectic approach, borrowing techniques from other methods to enhance their own teaching. Specific breathing and relaxation techniques described here will be discussed fully in chapters 4 and 5.

Lamaze.   This is the most popular technique of childbirth preparation in the U.S. today, accounting for about four out of five prepared deliveries, or well over two million births a year. ASPO (American Society for Psychoprophylaxis in Obstetrics)/Lamaze, the organization founded in 1960 to promote the Lamaze method, has accredited more than 10,000 teachers since it began training teachers in 1965, according to Dr. Francine Nichols, ASPO's certification project director. ASPO-certified teachers teach more than 150,000 series of childbirth classes each year.

To enter ASPO/Lamaze's certification program, a candidate must be a registered nurse, certified nurse-midwife, or physician, or must hold a bachelor's degree in a health- or education-related program that includes a supervised practicum. Most ASPO-certified childbirth educators (ACCEs) are nurses, but an ACCE might have a background in teaching, social work, counseling, or physical therapy.

ASPO/Lamaze's rigorous one- to two-year training program includes Lamaze class observations, intensive academic work in an approved university setting, labor and delivery observations, a teacher-training seminar, the writing of a detailed class syllabus, supervised student teaching, and standardized tests to assure competence in the subjects the ACCE will be teaching. ASPO teachers are required to observe some of their students' labors and deliveries, and to attend workshops and seminars in order to keep their certification current.

While Lamaze is popularly known as "the breathing"—anyone who has ever heard or seen Bill Cosby's routine on natural childbirth will never forget his parody of Lamaze breathing—the fundamental technique stressed in today's Lamaze classes is relaxation. "The breathing" today is simpler and slower than in its original formulation; it should be used only if a woman requires it to enhance her ability to relax. If she cannot relax during labor using her normal breathing, she may choose from a couple of simple patterns, adapting these to her own needs in order to increase her concentration on relaxing.

Because the body's natural response to stress is an interruption of normal breathing, substituting helpful breathing patterns can increase relaxation. Lamaze teachers encourage slow breathing throughout labor. But women may opt to breathe faster or use a more complex breathing pattern in order to cope with the contractions if they get increasingly painful. A number of comfort measures and attention-focusing techniques can be added to the rhythmic breathing patterns to enhance their usefulness.

What distinguishes Lamaze training is its goal of active concentration based primarily on relaxation and supplemented by rhythmic breathing patterns. To aid their concentration, women are encouraged to direct their attention to a focal point, which may be an internal image, or something to look at, listen to, or feel, or a body movement. Their partners are also taught effective verbal coaching and massage techniques to reduce pain perception even further.

Because your mind can concentrate only on so many things at once, a positive focus on relaxation, breathing patterns, and other comfort measures should substantially reduce the amount of concentration you have available to focus on your pain. As a result, you'll experience less pain.

For many women, this active approach to pain relief seems just right. One expectant mother put it this way, "I think Lamaze is very compatible with my personality. I'm a doer, one who prefers to take action to ameliorate my problems. I think what I've learned in Lamaze will be helpful under whatever conditions prevail during labor and delivery."

Some critics suggest that Lamaze techniques are tension-producing, control-oriented, or mere distractions from labor. In *Essential Exercises for the Childbearing Year,* Elizabeth Noble describes the Lamaze approach as "dissociating and blocking out discomfort."

But Lamaze teachers disagree. Suzanna May Hilbers, a longtime Lamaze teacher and former member of the ASPO/Lamaze faculty, claims that the goal of the Lamaze techniques is "not to dissociate from pain but to restructure it. We want people to confront, accept, and absorb their pain."

The Lamaze teacher helps students to separate "appraisal" (the recognition of pain that usually leads to tension and stress) from "alarm" (the manifestation of the fight-or-flight response), and to substitute for alarm positive measures that promote relaxation. These measures don't merely distract the mind from pain, but focus attention in a way that has been proven effective in reducing pain.

While some people may find attention-focusing synonymous with attempting to control labor, most Lamaze teachers don't see it this way. They may emphasize a woman's activity on her own behalf, but they prefer to see it as "active yielding" rather than controlling. A clinical psychologist who took Lamaze for the birth of her second child met her goal of avoiding medication during labor. She said afterward that "the nurse and obstetrician complimented me on my control. I think, though, that this was the opposite of what I was doing. I was trying to give up a need to control and to give over to my body's changes, without directing the birth."

Far from Lamaze's original formulation of childbirth without pain, most up-to-date Lamaze instructors don't promise a painless birth, but instead teach a variety of ways to cope with the pain that does exist. To most Lamaze teachers, pain is no longer the four-letter "p-word" to be eschewed in reverence to Dr. Lamaze. It's an important topic to confront honestly in class.

Lamaze classes usually include balanced information on medication and obstetric interventions. These procedures are presented along with their pros and cons rather than endorsed as routines or condemned as evils to be avoided under any circumstances. Most Lamaze teachers call what they teach "prepared childbirth" to emphasize a major point: that with preparation a woman will be able to make informed decisions about her own birth, including the choice of whether or not to take painkilling medication (see chapter 18).

Lamaze classes usually begin toward the end of pregnancy, though in many areas, early-bird classes are available. Since the original publication in 1967 of Elisabeth Bing's *Six Practical Lessons for an Easier Childbirth,* Lamaze classes have traditionally included six two- to two-and-a-half-hour sessions. Many teachers teach a slightly longer series, and some offer an abbreviated series for review couples. A full series may feature fewer but longer lessons, say four three-hour sessions, five two-and-a-half-hour sessions, or even a weekend intensive course. Plan on 12 hours of instruction as a minimum to be prepared in the Lamaze method.

Lamaze classes may take place in a variety of settings: hospitals, instructors' homes, churches, synagogues, and community centers. Class sizes and fees vary widely by location, but classes over 12 couples should include assistants to help check your progress.

Because Lamaze has become a household word and it is not patented, anyone can teach so-called "Lamaze" classes. Classes not taught by an ASPO/Lamaze-certified childbirth educator may or may not be designated by a lower case "l" for "lamaze." If you would like to know whether your Lamaze teacher has undergone a demanding training program, be sure to ask about her preparation and professional affiliation before you sign up for class.

Dick-Read's Natural Childbirth.   Grantly Dick-Read theorized that fear of the unknown caused a woman in labor to be tense, and that this unnecessary muscular tension led to much of the pain of labor. Indeed, the British doctor's formulation of the fear/tension/pain triad remains a cornerstone for just about every type of childbirth education taught in this country today. In addition, an American foundation to promote natural childbirth bears Dick-Read's name (see Resources).

Bradley's Husband-Coached Childbirth.   Husbands are expected to go into the delivery room today, but in 1947 when Dr. Robert Bradley began encouraging their attendance at births, husband-coached childbirth was considered outlandish. Dr. Bradley, an early follower of Grantly Dick-Read, was puzzled by some aspects of the Dick-Read method, primarily the use of panting breathing in labor and the fact that Dick-Read positioned himself at the head of the bed, ignoring the woman's husband. Bradley believed that the husband, not the obstetrician, should be at the center of the woman's childbirth experience. Bradley also thought that women should breathe abdominally throughout labor, speeding up their respiration naturally as their contractions progressed.

Growing up on a farm, Bradley had observed animals' instinctive knowledge of painless birth; his goal became to teach women through training and practice to do what animals did by instinct. He is forthright in calling his method "natural," not "prepared," childbirth because "the term 'natural' implies the way it is done in nature. . . .

[Our] fundamental goal is totally unmedicated pregnancy, labor, and birth."

According to Marjie Hathaway, director of the Academy of Husband-Coached Childbirth, about 1,200 certified Bradley teachers currently offer classes in almost every state. Teachers tend to be parents who have had a Bradley-style birth, though occasionally obstetric nurses are accepted into the training. The teacher education takes nine months and includes book reports, hospital surveys, and surveys conducted by the La Leche League, an organization for nursing mothers; a four-day, three-night workshop conducted by Marjie Hathaway and her husband, Jay; provisional teaching; and a final written exam. Like ASPO-certified Lamaze instructors, Bradley teachers are required to keep their certifications current.

Bradley classes for expectant parents last for twelve weeks (usually two hours per class). Many are taught by married couples, and class size is typically kept quite small. "A good class is five or six couples," says Marjie Hathaway. "Eight couples is a large class, and we'd be nervous at ten couples. We think small classes are important to good learning. Bradley teachers aren't affiliated with hospitals, so most teach in their own homes."

What do couples learn in a Bradley class? The Bradley method emphasizes relaxation and an inward focus. Many different types of relaxation are taught so that the laboring woman can use what relaxes her best. Unlike Lamaze classes, Bradley classes do not teach specific breathing patterns; instead, they prescribe a style of conducting labor that encourages a woman to relax as though she were sleeping.

According to Dr. Bradley, a woman's needs during labor are: darkness and solitude; quiet; physical comfort—aided by pillows that help the woman to assume the side-lying position; relaxation; abdominal breathing with mouth open; and closed eyes.

Bradley teachers acknowledge that labor hurts and they stress acceptance of pain. But Bradley instructor Rivka Willick says, "The safest birth for most women is unmedicated. Although there is a small percentage of women who need help, even they should have the least amount of medical intervention necessary."

The Academy of Husband-Coached Childbirth sets a goal of 90 percent unmedicated births; since some Bradley teachers are working in areas of the country where medicated births are the norm, Marjie Hathaway estimates an 86 percent rate of unmedicated births to Bradley-trained couples across the country. "In my own class," she says, "I get about 96 percent unmedicated births." The academy does not require the teachers to maintain a certain percentage of unmedicated births, but, according to Hathaway, "We encourage the teachers and we feel it's a possibility."

One mother who chose Bradley classes for her birth says, "I wanted to shoot for an unmedicated birth and to concentrate on what was happening in labor rather than dissociating myself from it. I also liked the fact that the Bradley teacher gave more classes and really stressed nutrition."

Fees for Bradley classes are set by the individual instructors. According to Marjie Hathaway, some Bradley teachers are so enthusiastic that they teach for no fee at all. She continues, "We encourage our teachers to charge a decent amount of money for what they're doing. But they're not in it for the money. They've had a Bradley birth themselves and thought it was wonderful, and they want to share it with other people."

Informed Homebirth/Informed Birth & Parenting. Since 1977, Informed Homebirth/Informed Birth & Parenting (IH/IBP) has certified nearly 2,000 teachers from the United States, Canada, and several foreign countries. Founded by author and midwife Rahima Baldwin to train homebirth teachers, IH/IBP expanded its role in 1981 to reach out to parents selecting hospital and birthing center deliveries. A typical IH/IBP course consists of seven classes.

Baldwin, president of IH/IBP, says that most of the teachers her organization certifies "teach privately rather than work for a doctor or hospital. As independent childbirth educators, they are free to emphasize true consumer awareness of choices in childbirth."

Like Bradley teachers, IH/IBP instructors teach slow relaxation breathing and specifically eschew the patterned breathing typically taught in Lamaze classes. Baldwin takes an eclectic approach to other pain-relieving strategies, emphasizing that there is no "right" way to have a baby and no method that is doomed to fail.

Teachers, preferably women who have given birth, may receive provisional certification either through correspondence or via attendance at a two-and-a-half-day training workshop held at various locations throughout the United States. Most IH/IBP teachers complete the requirements for full certification within one year. Full certification requires mastering a reading list, taking a course in infant CPR, and receiving positive evaluations from six couples. Teachers renew their certification annually by attending an all-day continuing education workshop and by critiquing a new book in the field. Teachers set their class fees independently.

The Gamper Method.   Though her name is not a household word as is Bradley's or Lamaze's, Margaret Gamper was a true pioneer in American childbirth education. A registered nurse in Chicago, Mrs. Gamper read Grantly Dick-Read's book in 1946 and became convinced that relaxation training could help her doctor's obstetrical patients. By 1949, Gamper's classes were written up in Chicago newspapers and she had produced America's first natural childbirth film. In 1955 she took the unprecedented step of leaving her employer to set up her own practice in childbirth education, and she has been teaching and training childbirth educators since then.

Margaret Gamper's method is based on Grantly Dick-Read's ideas and on the techniques she learned in her own training in Swedish massage and physical therapy. Gamper's additions to the Dick-Read method are two unique breathing techniques to lift the abdominal wall off the uterus during contractions, and a very basic, easy-to-learn relaxation technique based on yawning.

While Gamper method classes are easiest to find in the Midwest, Mrs. Gamper has been certifying teachers in her method since 1983 through a cooperative program at Loyola University in Chicago. To be certified as an instructor in the Gamper method, one must be a registered nurse or physical therapist, or have a medical background, or audit an obstetrics and gynecology course at a nursing school. A bachelor's degree is not a necessity; Mrs. Gamper believes that you don't have to have a bachelor of science degree to teach mothers how to have babies. She says, "I like my instructors to be down-to-earth and not to use extensive medical language." Basic training for Gamper teachers involves a three-day workshop at Loyola and about two years of follow-up training, much of it accomplished by correspondence.

Gamper classes begin in the fourth or fifth month of pregnancy, meeting at first biweekly, and then weekly, until the end of the eighth month, for a total of ten classes. Class size is limited to a maximum of 12 couples and class fees vary by location.

Sheila Kitzinger's Psychosexual Method.   A British childbirth educator and prolific author, Sheila Kitzinger originated what she calls the psychosexual method of childbirth. This method stresses birth as a profound psychological and sexual experience for a woman.

In *The Complete Book of Pregnancy and Childbirth*, Kitzinger says that her ideas about birth grew out of Dick-Read's and Lamaze's methods, with contributions from psychoanalytic theory and social anthropology. Like Dick-Read, Kitzinger emphasizes relaxation that puts a laboring woman more in tune with her body. Like Lamaze, Kitzinger suggests several breathing patterns for labor, each calibrated to the intensity and rhythm of the contractions. Kitzinger specifically developed two methods of relaxation: touch relaxation, and Stanislavsky techniques of imagining the contrasting sensations of bodily tension and relaxation (see pages 60 and 63).

Though no American organization specifically teaches the Kitzinger method, childbirth educators of every philosophy have been heavily influenced by her work for more than two decades. Most childbirth teachers integrate Kitzinger's techniques and approach into their own teaching.

Hospital-Sponsored Classes.   As childbirth education has become more popular, hospitals and even obstetricians' groups have begun offering their own prepared childbirth classes. According to the American Hospital Association's 1989 Survey of Obstetric and Newborn Services, more than 89 percent of responding hospitals answered "yes" to the question, "Does your hospital sponsor a class to prepare people for the delivery process?"

Hospital-sponsored classes are frequently taught by maternity nurses employed by the hospital. These classes often cost less than privately-sponsored ones and they can certainly familiarize you with the setting where you'll be giving birth. But hospital-sponsored classes may not always be such a great bargain. The classes tend to be large and they may devote little class time to practicing prepared childbirth techniques.

Some people find, too, that hospital-sponsored classes don't always present consumer issues forthrightly. One mother who took both hospital-sponsored and private childbirth classes says, "I never really learned what my options were from the hospital class. I certainly learned the hospital's routines for birth, but the teacher never presented the pros and cons on controversial issues."

Sandy Sheagren, a nurse who set up the prepared childbirth classes at Lutheran General Hospital in Park Ridge, Illinois, agrees that "the independent instructor can be more consumer-oriented than a hospital instructor can. Hospital classes may have 15 couples or more. Teachers employed by the hospital don't tell people as often about refusing procedures, and they can't be as strong about taking one side of an issue versus another."

Don't assume that just because a childbirth course is taught in a hospital or doctor's office its teacher must be a hired gun. Sheagren, for example, now teaches for a large group practice, but she considers herself an independent instructor because her students pay their fees directly to her. She says, "I teach anything I want to and I don't feel restrained or constrained."

The nurses who teach the prepared childbirth course sponsored by your hospital may be certified by a national organization such as ASPO/Lamaze or ICEA. More likely, however, they received a brief training in-house or perhaps a three-day seminar offered by Childbirth Education Specialists. If you're thinking of taking your hospital's prepared childbirth course, don't be hesitant to ask about the teacher's qualifications, training, and philosophy, just as you would screen an independent childbirth instructor.

Eclectic Methods. Many childbirth teachers combine elements of different methods, based on extensive reading, attendance at workshops, and observations of what seems to work for women in labor. As Margaret Gamper says, "All the childbirth methods have a lot of merit."

Since 1982, the International Childbirth Education Association (ICEA), an umbrella organization which supports family-centered childbirth, has been certifying eclectic childbirth educators. ICEA does not demand or even suggest any one particular method of teaching. Kimberly Dungey, administrator of ICEA's certification program, says, "One thing that attracts a lot of people is that we certify teachers in a philosophy rather than a method. Training to be an ICEA-certified childbirth educator is open to anyone who supports the ICEA philosophy of 'freedom of choice based on knowledge of alternatives.'"

ICEA certification requires the mastery of a core of knowledge, the teaching of a supervised series of classes, labor and delivery observations, and a standardized examination. ICEA's training takes two years and includes requirements for periodic recertification in order to ensure that teachers have up-to-date information and skills. As independent practitioners, ICEA-certified childbirth educators (ICCEs) set their own class fees, class sizes, and teaching locations.

Many childbirth books emphasize one or another aspect of preparation for childbirth in order to come up with a new slant on childbirth preparation. Author Gail Sforza Brewer, for example, developed a method she calls "cooperative childbirth." Eschewing Lamaze breathing patterns as energy-consuming and exhausting, Brewer says the basis of the cooperative method is to "cooperate with the powerful sensations of labor rather than trying to overcome, deny or disregard them." In *Nine Months, Nine Lessons*, Brewer emphasized staying relaxed in order to avoid painkilling drugs during labor. Wellpropped on at least five pillows, the pregnant woman practices relaxing while her partner simulates labor contractions by squeezing her muscles, a technique also taught in many other types of childbirth classes.

Instinctive Methods. In recent years, several books have been published that take a psychological, introspective approach to childbirth preparation. Uniformly critical of patterning breathing to ease labor pain, the authors stress a woman's acceptance of the pain of birth as a crucial element in her growth as a human being. Elizabeth Noble's *Childbirth with Insight*, Claudia Panuthos's *Transformation Through Birth*, Gayle Peterson's *Birthing Normally*, Michel Odent's *Birth Reborn*, and Janet Balaskas's *Active Birth* do not teach a method of childbirth so much as encourage a woman to look within to find her own resources for helping herself during birth.

Janet Balaskas, for example, writes, "Active birth is natural and instinctive. It is the way a woman, left to her own devices, will behave during labor. In preparing a woman for an active birth, my aim is to help her get in touch with her own birth-giving instincts."

In *Birth Reborn*, French doctor Michel Odent described how he fashioned his maternity unit in Pithiviers, France, to preclude any need for traditional childbirth education. At Pithiviers, wrote Odent, "we have almost nothing to teach . . . in the conventional sense of 'childbirth education' and . . . we reject entirely its prescriptive aspects." Odent, who currently attends home births in London, has recently published a new book called *Water and Sexuality*, in which he writes, "One simply cannot help an involuntary process; one can only disturb it."

Special Classes. Classes may be available in your area for vaginal birth after cesarean or for home birth. Consult the Resources section at the end of this book for organizations such as ICEA that can let you know where such specialized classes might be available.

Choosing Your Childbirth Class and Instructor

In choosing which method of childbirth preparation suits you best, you may find it helpful to decide how much time you are willing to spend on classes. Gamper or Bradley classes tend to have more sessions than Lamaze classes.

You should also consider how you feel about medication and

other interventions during birth. If you prefer little or no medication, seek out a teacher who will stress consumer awareness and spend a significant portion of class time practicing effective coping strategies for labor. You may be disappointed in a hospital-sponsored class that advertises the benefits but neglects to mention the risks of obstetric anesthesia.

On the other hand, if you're fairly certain you would like anesthesia for birth, you might appreciate a hospital-based class or an independent class with a balanced approach to obstetric intervention. You could feel uncomfortable in a class whose teacher is fervently committed to unmedicated birth.

To find an instructor, ask your birth attendant, look up "childbirth education" in the yellow pages, consult the childbirth organizations listed in the Resources section of this book, or use the expectant mother/new mother grapevine. One new mother learned that "when you're pregnant, people love to give you advice. I got my childbirth educator's name from a complete stranger who overheard me discussing birth with a friend at the health food store."

If acquaintances recommend their childbirth teacher to you, find out what they liked about their instructor. Were the classes interesting? Did they learn what they needed to know? Was the information accurate and up-to-date? Were the class handouts of high quality?

When you call to speak to a prospective instructor, you are hiring a professional, so don't be embarrassed to ask about professional qualifications. If your teacher has been certified by a national organization, you can be assured that she has had a rigorous training and has passed a standardized exam. You may want to know how long she has been teaching and how she keeps her information current. For example, does she attend workshops and conferences, subscribe to journals, read current books about birth, and attend the births of some of her clients? What are her beliefs about birth and her goals for the class?

If you are interested in specific topics, find out whether your class will cover them. Or, you can ask to be referred to another source of information.

Of course, you'll want to know practical things like meeting times, location and frequency of classes, fee, average class size, and an overview of what you'll be learning. More than a few women have been disappointed by the limited amount of time actually spent practicing prepared childbirth techniques in their classes. Many topics dealt with in lectures could be adequately covered through handouts, leaving sufficient time to practice pain-relieving techniques. Find out in advance what percentage of class time will be spent in practice.

If you have time, visit a childbirth class to see how well the teacher's style and philosophy mesh with your own. Most teachers are happy to be observed and will be impressed with your intelligent consumerism . . . particularly if you choose to enroll with them after all your diligent research!

Taking prepared childbirth lessons can give you great confidence in your ability to handle the powerful sensations of birth. Whatever method and instructor you select, you'll learn many practical ways of helping yourself during labor. The next chapters will cover the prepared childbirth techniques of relaxation and breathing in great detail, as well as a host of other techniques and aids that may be new to you.

4
Letting Labor Happen:
Relaxation

Virtually every method of preparation for childbirth emphasizes relaxation as the primary technique for keeping you comfortable during labor. That's because the more relaxed you can be during labor, the less your labor will hurt.

People feel more pain when they're tense. Try holding your whole body tense for ten or fifteen seconds. It hurts, doesn't it? If you spent your labor gritting your teeth and anticipating the next painful contraction, you'd be in considerable unnecessary pain because of your "grit and bear it" approach.

"Pain in childbirth," says Dr. Marlene Eisen, a clinical psychologist and hypnotherapist, "is just like that little Chinese puzzle you stick your two fingers into. If you pull hard, it tightens on your fingers and you can't get it off. If you move your fingers together and relax into it, it just falls right off. If you pull away from your labor pain and tighten up your muscles, that just creates increasing pain. But if you relax with it, the whole body system flows and it doesn't hurt nearly as much."

Tension in your voluntary muscles deprives the uterus of needed oxygen; this only compounds your pain. What's more, labor lasts longer when you're tense because high levels of tension can prevent your contractions from opening up the cervix.

Relaxing, on the other hand, reduces the tension that produces so much unnecessary pain. When you relax during labor, you put yourself in harmony with your body's work. Physical relaxation produces a calm mind, which allows you to adjust to the process of birth rather than fight it. Learning to relax helps assure that you do not add to the pain and length of your labor.

Relaxation works not only as a powerful positive focus for your attention during labor. It also helps you conserve energy to push the baby out. Unnecessary tension just wastes your energy and makes you too exhausted to participate.

In addition, relaxation enhances the effectiveness of every other method of pain relief. Women who relax during labor use significantly less pain medication; they also rate labor as a much more positive experience.

This chapter will give you many suggestions about working relaxation awareness and practice into your daily routine. When you give birth, you'll be glad you learned and practiced relaxation. One woman said, "It seemed our Lamaze teacher spent too much time on relaxation techniques during the class. But at the delivery when I was able to relax so thoroughly, we definitely saw the value."

Getting Started

You probably already have some idea of your body's reactions to stress and what helps you relax. Some people characteristically experience tension in the forehead and neck; others grit their teeth. Perhaps you feel tension in your chest, shoulders, or face. Do you get headaches when you're under stress? Does your stomach bear the brunt of your tension? As you learn to relax, try to pay extra attention to those parts of you most sensitive to stress. Try, too, to be aware of these trouble spots during the day so you can quickly release tension and go through your life more comfortably.

Give some thought to what enables you to relax. Perhaps it's a warm bath or making love with your husband, or lying in bed for a while before you fall asleep. Can you remember the wonderful feeling of heavy softness in all your limbs when you were fully relaxed? If you don't know what it feels like to be fully relaxed, don't worry; you can learn how. It may help to begin by looking at and feeling the limbs of a fully relaxed person—your partner, perhaps, as he sleeps— to feel just how heavy and limp you will be when you relax. You'll also want to have your partner's help to let you know how well you're progressing as you learn the skill of relaxing your body.

Most people find that they begin to release tension as soon as they start to slow down their breathing. It is particularly the exhaled breath—as in a sigh or a yawn—that brings on sensations of peace and restfulness. We'll talk much more about breathing in chapter 5.

Begin your relaxation practice in a very quiet atmosphere, but progress as you get more adept so that you are able to relax even in a noisy environment. You'll also want to start your relaxation practice in the most comfortable position you can think of. For pregnant women, this may be in a side-lying position, perhaps your sleeping position, with your head, chest, and upper arm supported on one pillow, and your upper leg supported on another. Extra pillows can be used wherever you need them, such as under your hip or abdomen. The guiding principle of comfort here is to allow the pillows to take the weight of your whole body. Each limb needs to be supported and each limb should be somewhat bent.

Perhaps you'd prefer to sit in a comfortable chair or recliner, your arms and hands resting on the arms and your legs resting on a hassock in front of you. If you have a beanbag chair, try that, or relax in bed, sitting up, with pillows supporting your slightly bent arms and legs. Don't scrimp with the pillows—just think of Cleopatra on her barge and treat yourself like a queen!

Once you are able to relax in any of the above positions, progress to practicing in a regular chair. Let your head and arms rest on a pillow placed on a table in front of you. When you understand the principle of relaxation, you'll begin to be aware of moments when you're tensing unnecessarily, and you'll be able to relax while you're going about your daily tasks.

For example, can you relax your arms, shoulders, and face when you are standing? When you drive your car or work at a desk, which muscles do you need to use and which can be relaxed? Learning to be aware of muscle tension and to ease it can help you to avoid expending unnecessary energy. This will come in handy as you move around during labor.

Working with Your Partner

You can improve your ability to relax merely by focusing your awareness on your body's sensations and the contrast between tension and relaxation. However, most women find it tremendously helpful to get feedback from their husband or labor partner to let them know if they are truly letting go of tension. As you practice, your partner should learn how you feel and look when you are tense and when you are relaxed. He can also discover the most effective ways of helping you relax by his voice and touch.

Your partner is a living biofeedback machine that lets you know what he sees and feels. When he checks to see if you're relaxed, he'll look at you for visible signs of tension: a furrowed brow, a clenched jaw or fists, lifted shoulders, or curled toes. He'll touch your limbs to feel if your muscles are soft (relaxed), or hard (tensed). He'll lift your limbs gently to see if you feel heavy, loose, and relaxed. If he supports you completely when he lifts you, you won't grow tense out of fear that he'll drop you.

If you do become tense, he should encourage you by saying, "Give me the weight," or "Let me hold it." He can massage you (see Touch Relaxation, below). He can also use words or catchphrases to help you relax, such as: *soft, warm, loose, heavy, let go, release, jello, pudding, limp noodle, rag doll.*

If you have trouble releasing in practice, your partner should try holding your tense limb up in the air until you begin to get tired and start to drop it. When you begin to let go, even a little, he should give you immediate feedback: "There, you did it just now, did you feel that?" Relaxation flows out toward the ends of your limbs. If you're not able to relax your arms, your partner should start at your hands and work upward until you can relax all the way to your shoulders.

Trained instruction can help you develop these skills, so both you and your partner will know exactly what you're striving for. Ask your childbirth educator for extra help if you need it.

Your partner will be necessary for some of the following techniques, while you can do others on your own. During labor, of course, your partner will be indispensable for helping you to maintain your relaxation under stress.

Relaxation Techniques

You can use many different techniques to promote relaxation. The ones described below differ from each other in several ways. Some keep your mind occupied, while others encourage a more passive letting-go. Some suggest that you tense or stretch before you relax, while others go directly for the relaxed feeling. Some require external help, like a partner or a tape recorder, while others can be done completely by yourself. Some you'll practice in your prepared childbirth class and some you'll learn on your own. If nothing here helps you feel relaxed, you may want to try a few lessons in biofeedback (see chapter 12). Biofeedback gives you instantaneous information on whether your muscles are relaxing.

Learning to relax is like learning to ride a bicycle. Once you know the feeling, you'll be able to produce it whenever you need it.

Progressive Relaxation. Dr. Edmund Jacobson originated this method of tensing and releasing muscle groups all over the body. The purpose of tensing the muscles is merely to feel the contrast when you release them or "go negative." The release—relaxation—is the important part of this practice; it's the opposite of holding tension in the muscles. According to Jacobson, it takes many sessions to learn to relax every single part of the body.

As you contract and release your muscles, try to notice if your muscles tense up in pairs or groups. As Dr. Jacobson wrote in *How to Relax and Have Your Baby*, "When an arm or other part of the body is really relaxed, other parts tend to relax with it. The relaxation spreads. But if a part is tense, other parts tend to become tense also." When you tighten the muscles of your arms, do you feel yourself clenching your jaw at the same time? Becoming aware of these unconscious pairings is a good first step to learning conscious release. Once you learn how to relax, you can skip the tensing up part and go directly for release (see Passive Relaxation, page 59).

You may want to have your partner read this exercise to you; or, you can record it for yourself on a cassette tape. Be sure to read the exercise very slowly, leaving sufficient time to feel the relaxation.

INSTRUCTIONS

Assume a comfortable reclining position, making sure that all your limbs are supported and slightly bent and that you are not lying flat on your back. Start to become aware of your breathing, slowing down and relaxing more on each exhaled breath. Allow your eyes to close. . . .

Wrinkle your forehead, lifting your eyebrows as high as you can, and hold for a few seconds. Release, and feel the tension flowing from your forehead and scalp. . . . Now close your eyes tightly and wrinkle your nose. Hold it for a few seconds, and let go, and feel the tension flowing out of your face. . . . Purse your lips and clench your teeth together. Hold for a few seconds. Now release the tension and feel your jaw drop and your tongue rest loosely in your mouth. . . . Push your head down toward your chest and hold for a few seconds. Relax. . . .

Now shrug your shoulders up toward your ears and hold for a few seconds. As you release, feel the tension leaving your neck and upper back. . . .

Clench your fists tightly and feel the tension in your hands. Hold for a few seconds. Now release the tension and allow your hands to relax. . . . Now tense your arms all the way to the shoulders, hold for a few seconds, and relax. . . .

Arch your back for a few seconds. Now release. . . . Tighten your abdominal muscles and hold for a few seconds. Let go. . . . Now tense your buttocks, hold, and release. . . .

Tighten your feet, pulling your toes up toward your knees. Hold for a moment. Relax your feet. . . . Tense your legs all the way up from your feet to your hips. Hold for a few seconds. Now, relax, and feel the tension flowing out of your feet.

Breathe slowly, releasing any residual tension on each exhaled breath. Bring your attention to any part of your body that feels tight or uncomfortable, and release it, tensing first, if necessary. . . . Take time to enjoy this relaxed state, noting the relaxation in your muscles now that you have let go of all tension. Your muscles feel limp and heavy, warm and comfortable. . . . Enjoy this good feeling for a few minutes. When you are ready to get up, stretch your arms and legs, take a deep breath, and open your eyes. Always get up slowly so you won't become dizzy.

Physiologic Relaxation.   Laura Mitchell, a British physiotherapist, based her relaxation method on the fact that muscles usually work in groups. When one group works, the opposite group relaxes; in order to relax muscles that are usually tense, you merely need to work the opposite group of muscles. The method, which Mitchell describes in her book *Simple Relaxation*, relies on direct orders to the muscles, and specifically eschews fanciful thoughts and meditation. Rather than tensing and releasing your muscles, as in the previous exercise, you will be doing muscle work—stretching—followed by resting and registering the feeling of ease.

To practice physiologic relaxation, assume a comfortable position, with head and limbs supported. As with the previous exercise, you may want to have the instructions read to you or taped for playing back.

INSTRUCTIONS

Pull your shoulders toward your feet. Stop and rest. Register this new position of ease. Your neck may feel longer.

Push your upper arms slightly away from your sides. Let your arms rest on something that supports them. Slide them along their support away from your body, moving at your shoulder joints. Now gently open the angle at your elbows by moving your forearms along their support away from your upper arms.

Stretch your fingers and thumbs out so that they are long. Stop and rest. Feel your fingers resting on their support, especially your heavy thumbs.

Turn your hips outward by rolling your kneecaps out toward the sides. Stop. Now adjust the position of your knees until they feel comfortable. Stop and rest. Feel the position. Push your feet away from your face, bending at the ankle. (Do this slowly and carefully to avoid getting cramps in your calf.) Feel your heavy feet dangling.

Breathe in and out through your nose at a slow rate. As you breathe in, feel your abdomen expand. As you breathe out, feel your ribs fall inward and downward.

Push your body against its support. Stop and rest. Feel the support holding your weight. Push your head into the support. Stop and rest. Feel the weight of your head resting on the support.

Drag your jaw downward. Feel your upper and lower teeth separated, your jaw heavy, and your lips loose. Press your tongue downward in your mouth. Feel your upper eyelids resting gently over your eyes. Think of the area just above your brows and imagine smoothing it out with a hand, then continuing into your hair, over the top of your head, and down to the back of your neck.

You may want to repeat the whole sequence, perhaps going a little faster. Now, choose what to think about, perhaps a happy memory, a song, a poem, or a prayer.

Enjoy the results of your work. Before getting up, always stretch your limbs and yawn before returning slowly to your activities.

Passive Relaxation.   With this technique, you don't need to do any muscle work—contraction or stretching—before relaxing, as in the previous two techniques. The following instructions are adapted from David Bresler's book *Free Yourself from Pain.* Tape the instructions or ask your partner to read them to you at a very slow pace. Give yourself plenty of time to follow each one.

INSTRUCTIONS

Find a comfortable position, using pillows to make sure that all parts of your body are supported. Arrange not to be interrupted during this exercise.

Begin by focusing on your breathing. Notice how slow, rhythmic breathing helps you become more relaxed. . . . Let your body breathe according to its natural rhythm. Take a cleansing breath in through your nose and out through your mouth; this will be your message to your body that you are entering a state of deep relaxation. Whenever you take this breath, your body will get the message to relax.

Now, as you continue breathing slowly, allow your eyelids to close. Feel the relaxing sensation around your eyes, from the top to the bottom, the sides, the front, and the back. . . .

Continue to breathe slowly. Allow the feeling of relaxation to radiate from your eyes out to your forehead. . . to your scalp. . . all around the back of your head. . . to your ears and temples. . . to your cheeks and nose. . . to your mouth. . . . Now relax your jaw muscles, allowing your jaw to open slightly, so that any remaining tension can just flow away.

Remember to keep your breathing slow and rhythmic. Now, relax the muscles in your neck and allow the feeling of relaxation to radiate down into your shoulders. Feel how heavy your shoulders are as you let the muscles relax. . . .

Now let the relaxation radiate down to your arms, to your elbows, your forearms, your wrists, and your hands. . . . Take a moment to relax each of your fingers—thumb, index finger, middle finger, ring finger, and little finger. . . . When your hands and arms are completely relaxed, you might notice feelings of warmth, heaviness, tingling, or pulsing. . . . All these are your body's way of telling you that you're relaxed.

Continue breathing slowly and rhythmically. Now let the feeling of warmth and release extend down your chest and abdomen, radiating around your sides and ribs, as relaxation flows from your shoulder blades down your upper back, middle back, and lower back. Let all the muscles on each side of your spine go. . . .

Send this release down into your pelvis and allow your buttocks to let go. . . . Feel the sensation of warmth and release move down your thighs, to your calves. . . your ankles. . . your feet. . . and your toes. Take a moment to relax each toe—big toe, second toe, third toe, fourth toe, and little toe. . . . Remember to breathe slowly and rhythmically, enjoying the feeling of release, letting go a little more each time you breathe out. . . .

Now that you are relaxed, start from the top of your head and work down, checking to see how relaxed you are. If any part of your body isn't fully relaxed and comfortable, simply take a breath in, and send healing, nourishing oxygen to that area to release the tension and allow it to melt away. As you breathe out, imagine that you are blowing out, through your skin, any tension, pain, or discomfort.

When you inhale, bring healing oxygen in, and when you exhale, blow away tension and discomfort. Send your breath to help release any part of your body that needs to be more relaxed. With each breath, allow yourself to become twice as relaxed as you were before.

When you are fully relaxed, take a moment to enjoy the good feeling, experiencing warmth and well-being throughout your body. . . .

Remember your slow, rhythmic breathing. To end this exercise, tell yourself that you can reach a deep state of relaxation, whenever you wish, simply by taking the cleansing breath. . . .

Conclude the exercise now by taking the cleansing breath in through your nose and out through your mouth. Feel energized, with a powerful sense of well-being and comfort.

Touch Relaxation.   This must be practiced with a partner, whose hands should be warm and relaxed. In *The Complete Book of*

Pregnancy and Childbirth, Sheila Kitzinger writes, "You are going to contract different sets of muscles—especially those you tend to tighten under stress—noticing how you feel when they are tight. Your partner will watch carefully, and then will rest one or both hands over the area you have tightened. As soon as you feel the touch you should relax and allow yourself to feel as if you were flowing out toward the touch." Likening the sensation of uterine contractions to a very powerful touch inside you, Kitzinger suggests that learning to release to your partner's pressure will enable you to meet your labor contractions with release.

These instructions are adapted so that you may choose between touch and massage—some women like still pressure, while others prefer stroking—to relax your tensed muscles.

INSTRUCTIONS

Woman	*Partner*
Assume a comfortable semiseated position.	
Frown or grimace.	Place two fingers on each of her temples and gradually release the pressure as she releases tension. *or* Place your palms in the middle of her forehead above her brow and stroke away the grimace with a long, continuous stroke.
Raise your eyebrows until you feel your scalp tighten.	Make a cap of your hands and rest them firmly on the top and back of her head. Gradually release this pressure as she releases tension. *or* Massage her scalp as though you were giving her a luxurious shampoo.
Grit your teeth.	Put palms on both sides of her jaw and gradually release pressure. *or* Stroke your hands along either side of her jaw.

Raise your shoulders toward your ears.

Apply firm pressure on her shoulders and gradually release it as she relaxes.
or
Massage her shoulders.

Squeeze your shoulder blades together in back.

Rest your hands firmly on the front of each shoulder.
or
Massage her shoulders down toward her elbows, using your palms with a long, continuous stroke.

Make a fist and tighten your arms, one at a time.

Firmly stroke down each arm, one at a time, ending with a massage of her hand.

Tighten your abdominal muscles, pulling in your stomach.

Stroke the lower curve of her abdomen, one hand following the other.

Press your thighs together.

Place your hands on the outside of each leg. Firmly stroke downward.

Press your knees out.

Stroke down the insides of her legs.

Tighten your legs, one at a time, avoiding pointing your toes.

Stroke firmly down each leg from her hip, ending in a massage of her foot.

In a side-lying position:
Jut your chin out.

Place your hands on the back of her neck.
or
Massage the back of her neck.

Arch your back.

Put your hands on the small of her back and stroke both sides firmly from the center outward.
or
Stroke her back from her shoulders all the way down to her buttocks, one hand following the other, as though you were

	swimming down her back. (Stroke down the sides of her spine, not the middle.)
Tighten your buttocks.	Put your hands on her buttocks and release your touch as she releases tension.
	or
	Firmly massage her buttocks, as though you were kneading bread.

Stanislavsky Relaxation.   In this method of relaxation, you imagine different activities involving the muscles that would be used to perform them. It is described in Sheila Kitzinger's *The Experience of Childbirth*. First you note the tension, and then you deliberately release the muscles. You've probably already practiced this technique without knowing it. Are you ever aware of how your body tenses up while watching a particularly scary movie or television show? Next time you become aware of this reaction, see if you can consciously relax.

Two examples from Kitzinger's book follow. Before doing these (or any other relaxation exercises), get into a comfortable position.

INSTRUCTIONS

Imagine that you are pulling on tight jeans that are still damp from washing. Act the movements, and really feel the effort to get them up over your thighs, buttocks, the bulge in front and, at last, on up to the waist. Now you have to do up the zip at the side. Pull hard. Notice what is happening to your breathing. You know how painful it is when bare flesh catches in a zip, so do this very carefully. This is contraction of the abdominal muscles. And now: relax! Now *that* is abdominal relaxation! Once you are relaxed, notice the sensation. This is how the abdominal muscles will be throughout labor, as you do not need to use them then.

See a large six-story building in front of you and watch a fireman hoist a ladder and climb slowly to the top story. . . . Now watch him slowly coming down again. He is at the bottom. Rest your eyes.

In *The Experience of Childbirth* and in her many other books, Kitzinger has developed a variety of Stanislavsky exercises for imagining tension and release—for the feet, for the hands, and for the face. Perhaps you'll want to use her exercises, or you could create your own "scripts" to feel the contrast between muscle tension and relaxation. For example: Construct an unpleasant situation—you're alone in a cold room, say, and you hear mysterious noises. Build up the picture in your mind, and feel your body's tension. Then, construct a pleasant scene with all your senses and put yourself in the middle of it. Feel yourself relaxing now.

For other exercises using visualization as a help to relaxation, see chapter 13.

Yawn and Stretch Relaxation.   In *Preparation for the Heir Minded*, Margaret Gamper suggests that the relaxation techniques taught by other childbirth educators are unnecessarily complex, requiring considerable practice to do properly. Her method of yawn and stretch relaxation, on the other hand, couldn't be simpler to learn. Yawning causes your lungs to expand, stimulates your heart, and charges your blood with oxygen. It also brings on a natural stretch, making it a convenient exercise for your lungs, face, and muscles. You can do this relaxation technique anywhere, anytime.

INSTRUCTIONS

Make yourself comfortable on your couch or bed in your favorite position. Use one or two pillows to give yourself a soft luxurious feeling.

Start by tightening your shoulder muscles as you tuck your head in between them. Visualize how the turtle tucks his head into his shell; he can't raise the shell, but you can raise your shoulders.

Tense every muscle. Clench your fists as tight as possible and do not let go; tighten the muscles of your buttocks and legs. (Point your toes toward your nose.)

Hang on until you experience a tight, numb feeling in the hands, then let go all over, just like a bucket of molasses spilled in the hot sun. As you let go, yawn, not once, but again and again. Open your mouth if necessary to produce your yawn, wiggling your jaw from side to side as you slowly fill your lungs with air. Now exhale slowly. If the shoulders still feel tight, think of your shoulder blades as wings. Make them rotate a few times by rotating the elbows in a circle. Close your eyes as you yawn again. Let loose all over.

Part your lips in a faint Mona Lisa smile, just so the teeth and tongue are not touching. The tongue should rest loosely in your mouth; every muscle in your face should be relaxed.

The Relaxation Response.   Popularized by Dr. Herbert Benson, the "relaxation response" is a part of many different types of meditation techniques. All these techniques—Zen, yoga, and transcendental meditation, for example—elicit the same beneficial physiological changes: decreases in heart rate, blood pressure, and oxygen consumption. The relaxation response is simple to do and requires minimal instruction.

INSTRUCTIONS

Assume a comfortable position with the eyes closed.

Deeply relax all your muscles from your feet up to your face.

Become aware of your breathing, concentrating on a single word or phrase each time you exhale.

Keep a passive attitude and let yourself relax. Expect other thoughts to occur to you, but gently bring your concentration back to your focus each time you exhale. (Benson suggests the word "one," but you can pick your own word or phrase.)

Practice for about fifteen to twenty minutes, once or twice a day, at least two hours after eating.

When done, sit quietly for several minutes with your eyes closed; then open them slowly.

The techniques that follow assume that you are already able to relax. You may want to try them after you have had some practice in the relaxation techniques described above.

Active Relaxation.   Sometimes called neuromuscular release, controlled relaxation, or selective relaxation, this exercise is typically taught in Lamaze classes to test your ability to relax the rest of your body while one set of muscles is contracted. In practice sessions, the contracted muscles serve to simulate the contracting uterus, so that you can learn how to use your concentration to stay relaxed while you are in labor.

Your partner will tell you to contract a limb or limbs and then he will check the rest of your body for relaxation. He can check you by looking for visible signs of tension, by touching you to see if you feel soft and loose, or by lifting your limbs one at a time to feel for the heaviness and lack of resistance that characterize relaxation. He should, of course, never drop you or shake your limbs vigorously, but rather lift you gently at the joints, bearing your weight himself and rotating your limbs slightly to feel for relaxation. If you need encouragement, he can give this verbally or by massaging you (see Touch Relaxation, page 60).

After he checks the rest of your body (or after sixty seconds have gone by), he will tell you to release tension, stroking the previously contracted limbs, allowing you enough time to relax. His and your concentration should always be on relaxation, not on whether you are contracting your limbs well enough, just as in labor your concentration will be on relaxing yourself in order to let your uterus do its job. Although this exercise is hard at first, you will improve with practice; your partner should try it, too, so he can better appreciate what you are trying to do.

You may want your partner to rate you on a scale of 0 (not relaxed at all) to 5 (fully relaxed) each time you practice this exercise. Start with single limbs and simple combinations, before you work up to the more challenging ones.

INSTRUCTIONS

Assume a comfortable position, all limbs supported and slightly bent. Take a few minutes to relax your body. Breathe slowly and rhythmically.

Your partner gives you the signal to contract your left arm. He checks for relaxation in the rest of your body; then he touches or massages your left arm and tells you to relax it, checking to see that you do so. Progress from one-limb contractions to contracting both arms, both legs, the left side, the right side, and finally, to difficult combinations like "left arm and right leg."

Autogenic Relaxation.   Autogenic training is based on the idea that you can learn to exert control over unconscious and involuntary processes like your heartbeat and body temperature, thereby reducing stress. Developed by psychiatrist Johannes Schultz in Berlin in the 1930s, autogenic training requires that you be relaxed and in a state of passive concentration, so that you will allow the body changes of warmth, heaviness, calm heartbeat, regular breathing, relaxation, and alertness to happen. You may want to have a partner read the instructions, or make a practice tape for yourself.

INSTRUCTIONS

Relax in a comfortable position and begin by focusing on your breathing, slowing down to a comfortable pace. Picture each body part in your mind, and continue to maintain your slow, rhythmic breathing.

My right arm is warm.	Repeat three times, then move to left arm, right leg, left leg, trunk, repeating three times for each of these.
My right arm is heavy.	Repeat as above.
My heartbeat is calm and regular.	Repeat three times as you concentrate on feeling your heartbeat.
My breathing is calm and regular.	Repeat three times and continue regular breathing until you feel very relaxed.

My forehead is cool.

Repeat three times as you begin to feel relaxed and alert.

I am relaxed, at peace, and alert.

Repeat three times and enjoy the feelings.

Quickie Relaxation Techniques. You may not always have time to set up pillows and have an elaborate practice session for relaxation. The following three techniques may all be done on the spur of the moment and are very effective at promoting relaxation in a hurry.

Breathing Focus:
1. Sit comfortably. As you inhale, think "I am . . . ," and as you exhale, think "relaxed." Repeat several times, relaxing more with each breath.
2. With each inhaled breath, reach for tension somewhere in your body. As you exhale, release the tension. Repeat several times.
3. As you breathe in, think of taking in oxygen and energy. As you breathe out, release tension or pain. Repeat several times.

Yawn and Stretch Relaxation:
See page 64.

Tension Release:
Tense all the muscles in your body and release. Repeat twice. Then take ten slow breaths, relaxing more with each exhalation.

Because relaxation is so important, practice every day, with or without your partner. During labor, your practice will come in handy. "I could relax completely," says one mother. "I played 'rag doll' with my arms, using their absolute limpness to keep the rest of my body relaxed. Between contractions, Karl would lift my arm slightly, only to have it drop like a rock. I chose to drift into a fog at the end of each contraction, and my ability to do this gave me the energy I needed to concentrate intensely through the next one."

As you undoubtedly know, the ability to relax isn't important only for labor but comes in handy after the baby's born, too. In fact, it's a skill we all need to cultivate. Mental relaxation and physical freedom from tension and stress positively affect the function of your muscles, thoughts, and emotions. After you learn to relax to give birth, you'll be able to use what you've learned to improve the rest of your life.

5
Gentle Inspiration:
Breathing for Labor

Breathing during labor is a subject of heated controversy among childbirth educators. Some contend that women should not be taught breathing techniques, while others argue that learned breathing patterns are a powerful aid to relaxation.

At first glance, perhaps, the debate may seem pointless. After all, we all know how to breathe well enough to do it in our sleep; couldn't we be expected to be able to breathe properly through labor, another natural function of our bodies? Dr. Bradley said yes. If a woman is deeply relaxed during labor, he argued, she will breathe according to her body's needs without any instructions at all. Bradley teachers specifically advocate relaxed abdominal breathing, allowing the woman's needs to determine the rate and depth of each breath. They caution against teaching chest-breathing techniques because these may lead to tension and hyperventilation.

Lamaze teachers agree that relaxation is the essential ingredient for coping with labor. But they feel that learned breathing patterns add a positive attention focus that decreases pain and promotes relaxation. As one mother says, "Having the relaxation and breathing to concentrate on rather than the pain made all the difference in my labor. Rather than anticipating the next contraction in dread and fear, I was waiting for the next opportunity to do my breathing. There's a terrific psychology behind the whole idea."

Indeed, many experimental studies of pain have shown that a purposeful change in respiration—pacing breathing according to a rhythmic pattern—decreases the body's response to stress. Because breathing tends to speed up naturally as labor progresses, Lamaze teachers advocate practicing at a faster rate so you can feel confident and relaxed if you need to breathe faster during labor.

Even though it is usually more relaxing to slow down your breathing, at times in your labor a faster pace may help you manage better. Breathing faster can make you more alert and allow you to cope with the more painful contractions and not be overwhelmed by them. You'll be the best judge of how to pace your breathing when you're actually in labor, though practicing under conditions of stress can give you a good idea of how pacing will help you relax in labor.

How Labor Breathing Helps You

Breathing and relaxation work hand in hand. When you are very relaxed, your breathing tends to become calm and regular. When you are tense, deliberately slowing down your breathing can enable you to become more relaxed.

How you breathe provides an unmistakable message about how you are doing. If your breathing gets rapid and out of control, for example, your body hears the message that something is wrong. Your fight-or-flight response kicks in and you get the classic signs of anxiety: increases in blood pressure, heart rate, and muscle tension. If you calm your breathing down, on the other hand, your body gets the message that everything is all right, and tension quickly dissipates.

Maintaining a focus on your breathing forces you to concentrate on what is happening here and now rather than being anxious about what might happen in the future. Since breathing is a powerful focus for your attention, concentrating on calm breathing takes away some of your ability to focus on pain. Thus, calm breathing decreases your perception of pain at the same time that it increases your feeling of going with the flow. What's more, if you're breathing properly, you'll be getting a healthy dose of oxygen for you and your baby, and you'll be working with labor rather than against it.

Practicing Breathing for Labor

Whether you learn specific breathing patterns or merely wish to become aware of your breathing, try deliberately keeping your breathing calm and regular during simulated contractions. You can simulate contractions by asking your partner to apply firm pressure to certain parts of your body. Your childbirth educator can show your partner exactly where and how to grip your muscles. Some popular spots are: just above the knee, just above the elbow, the trapezius muscle in the shoulder (for "Star Trek" fans, the location for the "Vulcan death grip"), the Achilles tendon above the ankle, and the fleshy part of the inner thigh. Your partner should vary the peaks of the contractions, sometimes pressing very hard at the beginning and slowly decreasing, and sometimes building pressure gradually to a peak in the middle. It will help if you practice coping with different kinds of contractions through relaxation and breathing.

In *Essential Exercises for the Childbearing Year*, author and childbirth educator Elizabeth Noble recommends a cooperative stretch with your partner to prepare you to cope with the pain of labor. She writes, "The key to surrender is releasing on the *outward* breath, which is the natural relaxation phase of the respiratory cycle. Moaning and groaning also help, as sound is energy, and opening the mouth aids in opening the pelvis."

To do Noble's forward stretch with your partner, sit on the floor with your legs stretched out, the soles of your feet touching his, and your hands clasped together. If your pubic joint is too tender for this, move closer to your partner and press your soles against his calves. Straighten your knees and back, using a book to perch on, if necessary. As your partner leans back, keeping his arms straight, allow him to pull you forward slowly to your limit—the "edge of pain"—which you should feel along the insides of your thighs. Noble suggests releasing into this simulated contraction for a minute or two at a time. She warns, "Don't bounce or force this stretch. You are increasing your flexibility by *learning to let go*, not trying to pull yourself apart!"

To avoid your partner's having to inflict pain, you may prefer to hold an ice cube in a baggie or to stick your hand into ice water for practice instead.

Here are some other suggestions to aid your breathing practice:

■ Practice every day.
■ Practice coping with contractions in different locations—in the car, in the shower, walking around—and in different positions

you might assume during labor, noting how different positions make you feel.

- Practice when you get Braxton-Hicks contractions (see page 7).
- Try contractions of different lengths, from 30 seconds to 120 seconds long.
- Experiment with adding rhythmic movement, music, and self-massage to see how these affect your breathing and relaxation.
- Try making sounds as you exhale—humming, sighing, moaning, saying a mantra or phrase—and note how this affects you.
- Compare using an external focus of concentration (a picture, a flower, or your partner's face) to using an internal focus (a soothing image such as a wave rising and falling, a mantra or phrase, or counting) to see which you prefer.

Lamaze Breathing

In 1983 ASPO/Lamaze updated its breathing techniques to accommodate the widely varying individual needs of different women. Lamaze training once emphasized chest breathing. The current approach, on the other hand, eliminates all specifications of where the breathing should take place, and states merely that breathing for labor should be "a relaxed motion of the chest and abdomen." In fact, some women normally breathe with their chests and some breathe abdominally. What part of your anatomy moves with respiration also depends on your position.

It really doesn't matter whether you breathe into your chest or into your abdomen during labor. Women seem to be helped by instructions to do either type of breathing. Focusing on breathing calmly, rather than doing a certain type of breathing, will help you relax.

When you practice the breathing patterns described below, adapt them to suit your own style and comfort. To see if a breathing technique is working for you during labor, ask yourself the following questions:

- Is the breathing making me feel more relaxed?
- Am I getting enough air?
- Do I feel less pain?

The Cleansing Breath.   You'll take this breath at the beginning and end of each contraction in labor. Typically, it's suggested that you inhale the cleansing breath through your nose and exhale it through your mouth. The cleansing breath signals to you, your partner, and your birth attendants that you've begun a contraction. Through practice you can soon condition yourself to think "relax, focus, and breathe calmly" whenever you take this breath.

Some people prefer to call the opening breath a "greeting" or "organizing" breath and the closing one a "goodbye" breath that helps you take leave of the contraction. Whatever you choose, make it part of your practice and let it help you relax and focus on breathing.

Slow-Paced Breathing.   You can try this pattern when you need to concentrate on breathing to augment your relaxation. The suggested pace is about half your normal breathing speed. Since most people breathe about 12 to 18 times in a minute, you'll probably do slow breathing at about six to nine breaths per minute. Have your partner time you when you aren't looking to determine your typical breathing rate.

You'll accomplish slow-paced breathing with a relaxed motion of your chest and abdomen. You can breathe in and out your nose (most like normal breathing), in and out your mouth (if you have a stuffy nose), or in through your nose and out through your mouth (a learned technique that focuses your attention on your breathing).

Along with the breathing, you may want to try some accompanying strategies to focus your attention even more:

- Time the length of the contractions (your partner can do this by counting off fifteen-second intervals).
- Count to yourself as you breathe in and out.
- Focus on a soothing image.
- Repeat a calming phrase or mantra.
- Imagine your breath flowing into the parts of your body where your partner places his hands.
- Rock your body in time with the breathing.
- Get a massage or massage yourself.
- Hum or sigh with the breathing.

Stay with slow-paced breathing as long as possible. It's the most relaxing and energy-conserving of all the breathing techniques. If you can no longer relax with slow-paced breathing, try the next breathing technique.

Modified-Paced Breathing.   This breathing technique may be done at 24 to about 40 breaths per minute, about twice your normal rate. Faster breathing is alerting, and this may be useful for you at some point in labor.

But some women find that speeding up their breathing triggers an anxiety response, making them feel tense and nauseated. In addition, rapid breathing can be fatiguing. So speed up your breathing only if it helps you to cope better; and return to slow breathing whenever you can, perhaps after the peak of each contraction.

Like slow-paced breathing, you'll do this technique with a relaxed movement in your chest and abdomen, but you'll also use your intercostal (between the ribs) muscles more. This happens quite naturally, so don't worry about it. You needn't be concerned about detailed instructions on how to hold your lips or place your tongue. Just do whatever feels right and comfortable. Breathe in and out through your nose, your mouth, or a combination of the two.

When you are doing the modified-paced breathing, you'll probably be paying more attention to timing and focusing more intensely on maintaining a rhythmic pattern of breathing. You may want to accelerate and decelerate your rate of breathing, so that you breathe more quickly at the peak and slow down when the contraction eases. Of course, you can add other attention-focusing strategies, too, such as listening to faster-paced music, concentrating on counting or a mantra, making sounds with the breathing, or concentrating on an internal or external visual focus.

Patterned-Paced Breathing.   Patterned-paced breathing can be used to add a repetitive rhythm you may find calming at a stormy time during your labor. The rate is the same as modified-paced breathing (twice your normal respiratory rate), and you'll find your own method of breathing comfortably.

The patterning comes in when you intersperse the rhythm of breathing with a soft candle-blow every one to six breaths. This technique focuses your attention on counting and on varying your activity. Some women choose to do one breath/one blow at the peaks of the contractions, and gradually decrease to six breaths/one blow in the valleys.

You may prefer instead to have your partner show you a random pattern by indicating different numbers with his fingers. Perhaps you'll want to direct yourself in a predetermined pattern, like six breaths/one blow, five breaths/one blow, four breaths/one blow, and so on, down to one breath/one blow, and then back up again to six breaths/one blow. Some mothers like to pattern their breathing in response to the contraction and hold up fingers to show their partners how to breathe along.

As with the other patterns, imagery, sound, or rhythmic movement can also work with this breathing technique to keep you relaxed.

Many women find that it helps to keep their eyes open and focused on their partner at this time. One mother said, "My husband was my lifeline. I just focused on his eyes and followed his demonstration of the breathing."

Avoiding Hyperventilation.   If you breathe too quickly and deeply at the same time, you may throw off the balance of oxygen and carbon dioxide in your blood, a condition called hyperventilation. Hyperventilation often accompanies feelings of tension or panic. You can prevent it by doing two things: staying relaxed, with your shoulders dropped; and keeping the speed and depth of your breathing inversely related—that is, if you speed up, stay shallow, and if you get deep, slow down.

You'll know you're hyperventilating if you feel dizzy. You may also get an uncomfortable tingling in your fingers, your feet, and around your mouth. If you kept breathing this way, you would pass out briefly; then your system would automatically right itself and your symptoms would abate. But you don't need to pass out to get relief. You can alleviate the dizziness, tingling, and oxygen–carbon dioxide imbalance merely by correcting your breathing, breathing into tightly cupped hands or a paper bag, or by holding your breath for several seconds as soon as your contraction is over.

When childbirth instructors taught a very rapid rate of breathing (60 to 120 breaths per minute), critics claimed that women who breathed too quickly and deeply would hyperventilate to the point of depriving their babies of oxygen. But a study conducted in the 1960s showed that hyperventilation led to fainting before it affected the baby's blood gases. In other words, hyperventilation threatens *your* comfort, but it does not pose a serious risk to your baby. Practicing your breathing, particularly under simulated stress situations, can give you confidence about staying calm and not hyperventilating during labor.

Breathing to Control an Urge to Push.   If your baby's head has moved deeply into your pelvis, you may get an urge to push before your cervix is completely dilated. This reflex urge causes you to get a catch in your breathing as you begin to hold your breath or grunt involuntarily with the pushes. If your cervix were still tightly closed, premature pushing could cause you more pain and perhaps even swell your cervix shut.

If you feel like pushing, get checked by your doctor, midwife, or nurse. In the meantime, you can prevent yourself from giving way to the pushing urge by learning to blow rapidly and repeatedly as though you were quickly blowing out all the candles on your birth-day cake, one at a time (inhale-blow, inhale-blow, inhale-blow, etc.). If this makes you feel dizzy, practice blowing into tightly cupped hands.

Kitzinger Breathing.   As described in her many books, Sheila Kitzinger's breathing techniques resemble Lamaze breathing. Kitzinger adds a lovely touch, however. She suggests you learn the breathing pat-terns with your partner's hands on different parts of your body, bring-ing your breath right down to the level of his hands and relaxing as you feel his touch.

For "full chest breathing," Kitzinger's first technique, your partner holds his hands at your waist, on either side of your spine. For stronger contractions, "upper chest breathing" finds his hands on your upper back just below your shoulder blades. You breathe this way through parted lips, with a little sigh each time you exhale, floating over the top of the contraction as if you were going over the crest of a wave.

The "butterfly" technique, according to Kitzinger, is the shallowest breathing of all, centered in your mouth behind your cheeks, and done extremely rapidly. Save it for the very hardest contractions. As in Lamaze patterned-paced breathing, you emphasize one beat out of every so many breaths. Take special care not to breathe too deeply at this rapid rate.

Breathing for the Birth

For the last 30 years, obstetricians have been directing women to work hard at pushing their babies out, encouraging prolonged breath-holding and muscular effort. Childbirth educators contributed to this phenomenon by teaching women to take full, deep breaths and hold them for as long as possible while straining mightily to push. One of the reasons so much effort was necessary, of course, was the standard lithotomy position for birth. Lying flat on her back with her legs up in the air, a woman had to work hard to push her baby uphill around the pubic bone. Fortunately, the recent emphasis on more upright positioning for birth has lessened some of this unnecessary effort (see chapter 10).

As it turned out, all that forceful pushing wasn't only hard on the mother, it was bad for the baby, too. In the late 1970s Roberto Caldeyro-Barcia, a Uruguayan obstetrician and former president of the International Federation of Gynecologists and Obstetricians, demonstrated conclusively that prolonged bearing-down efforts with breath-holding led to decelerations of the fetal heart rate. They also prompted a pronounced drop in maternal blood pressure, thereby reducing the baby's oxygen. On the other hand, when women pushed spontaneously, according to their own efforts, they seldom pushed more than five or six seconds at a time and they avoided putting their babies at risk.

After Caldeyro-Barcia's results came out, childbirth educators began to advocate a more instinctive approach to pushing. Author Elizabeth Noble led the way by suggesting exhalation while pushing as a natural method of preventing excessive strain on the mother's circulatory system. Not only does a woman who pushes spontaneously experience less exhaustion and fewer blood pressure changes, she also breaks fewer blood vessels in her face and eyes, and she runs a lower risk of tearing her cervix and vagina. Her baby, too, is unlikely to experience oxygen deprivation during the pushing stage. Following Noble's lead, many prepared childbirth classes began to advocate exhalation as an alternative to the old hold-your-breath-for-as-long-as-you-can-and-push-like-hell approach.

A study published recently in the *Journal of Obstetric, Gynecologic and Neonatal Nursing* supports the instinctive approach to pushing. Thirty-one untrained first-time mothers simply received encouragement to do what came naturally when they felt like pushing. These women pushed for an average of only 45 minutes and all their babies got good Apgar scores. The women's pushing efforts grew longer and more numerous as the second stage progressed, but their pushes still came in short bursts, only about four to six seconds long, for a total of three to five pushes in each contraction. Most mothers took several breaths to punctuate their pushing efforts, and, three-quarters of the time, they released air as they pushed. If they held their breath to push, they rarely did so for more than six seconds.

Recall that you may get the urge to push before you are completely dilated. Interestingly, in the same study, women who began to push at eight or nine centimeters of dilatation experienced no problems with cervical laceration as long as the baby's head was engaged and in an anterior or transverse (sideways) position.

Or, you may not get the urge to push until you are several minutes into the second stage, when your uterus is ready to do its part of the job. Don't worry. Sheila Kitzinger has called this the "rest-and-be-thankful" part of labor. Once the uterus pushes your baby down onto the pelvic floor, where stretch receptors stimulate the release of oxytocin, you'll get an irresistible urge to bear down.

If the urge to push does not come within about 20 minutes after you're fully dilated, you might try squatting. Only squat, however, if your baby's head is engaged. If your baby's head is still high, squatting may delay your progress because it narrows the entrance to the pelvis while it enlarges the outlet.

You might also try pushing while seated on the toilet; gravity-enhancing positions tend to bring the baby's head down to where your bearing-down reflex will be set off. When this happens, you will know it—it's tremendous and irresistible, so get ready to work with it.

Urges to bear down come after the contraction begins, so take a cleansing breath or two at the start of the contraction to help you find your focus and relax. Round your back and relax the muscles around your vagina. Push as you feel the urge, either by holding your breath and bearing down, or by exhaling forcefully (grunting or groaning is the way most women instinctively do this). In between the urges to push, you may want to do modified-paced breathing (what Sheila Kitzinger calls "sheep's breathing")—a quick, light breath that helps you ride the contraction until your next urge to push. Don't hold your breath with the pushes for more than five or six seconds at a time unless you're specifically directed to because of a medical emergency that mandates your baby's immediate birth. Some women like to have their partners count off the seconds as they push.

The best thing you can do to lessen pain during this stage is to release the muscles around your vagina and allow your baby to come down. You may want to have your partner suggest that you "open" or "release," because this will remind you not to work against your own efforts by contracting the muscles of your pelvic floor. If you keep your mouth open, it seems to help you to remember to relax around your vagina.

Right before your baby is born, you can see in the mirror that his head no longer goes back in between your pushes. It stings when the baby's head distends your vaginal opening. Dr. Grantly Dick-Read called this feeling the "rim of fire." You may have prepared for this feeling by doing perineal massage (see chapter 8). At birth you can cope with it by breathing lightly in and out through your mouth or by candle-blowing. Your doctor or midwife will probably be directing you to relax and breathe lightly or blow at this point. Some attendants also use methods to enhance your comfort and prevent the need for an episiotomy (a small incision to enlarge the vagina before birth). For example, they may apply warm, wet compresses to your perineum (the skin between the vagina and anus) or they may encourage your perineum to stretch by giving you a soothing oil massage (see chapter 17).

To summarize, if your labor has proceeded normally, push only with your urges, breathing lightly in between the five- to six-second pushing bursts. While pushing, hold your breath if that feels right, or let your air out with a sustained groan, or a grunt if that works better for you. Be sure to relax yourself at the end of each contraction with several good cleansing breaths. As the baby's head begins to distend your vagina and you feel the burning sensation, follow your birth attendant's directions to breathe, blow, or push gently as the baby is born.

Remember that the urge to push may not come on for 10 to 20 minutes into the second stage and that it is often stimulated by more upright positions. Sometimes, however, the urge to push never comes, often because epidural anesthesia has failed to wear off (see chapter 18). If you wait until you feel like pushing, you'll work less hard and get a bigger reward for your efforts.

If for some other reason you must push without having the urge, you can adapt the pushing technique as follows: At the start of each contraction, take a couple of good cleansing breaths. On the third breath, hold it and bear down and out of the vagina, relaxing your pelvic floor muscles. Bear down in five- to six-second bursts until your contraction begins to fade away. Take two more cleansing breaths and relax deeply at the end of each contraction.

If your baby is in distress and needs to be born quickly, you may be encouraged to hold each push longer and not to take any breaths between your pushes.

Now that you've learned about different breathing patterns for labor, perhaps you'd like to try one that puts you in touch with your soon-to-be-born baby. Adapted from *Positive Pregnancy Through Yoga* by Sylvia Klein Olkin, this breathing exercise is called "Rock-the-Baby," and it should feel good, to you and your baby.

> Sitting comfortably in a relaxed position, exhale completely through your nose. Now relax your abdominal muscles and inhale through your nose, sending the air directly to your baby. When you're done inhaling (about five seconds), exhale smoothly and slowly (about five to eight seconds), tightening your abdominal muscles and hugging your baby as you do so.
>
> When you inhale, your abdomen moves forward and when you exhale it moves back, so you're actually rocking your baby back and forth. Try it five to ten times and see if your baby doesn't send you a little kick of gratitude for the extra oxygen and the soothing rocking motion.

Introduction to Chapters 6–16

You can relieve labor pain in a number of ways: by blocking nerve pathways, by overriding pain impulses with stronger sensations, by refocusing your thought elsewhere, by easing the muscle tension that promotes pain, and by reducing painful stimuli in your environment. Because so many different methods can ease labor pain, some of them will surely work for you.

Often the combination of a few different methods will be more effective than any one method used individually. So try a variety of techniques. Because women who previously have coped successfully with pain unrelated to childbirth seem to manage better during birth, employ methods that have worked for you in the past and in which you have confidence.

Your mind and body work as one, so it's hard to say that a method is strictly physical or psychological. In general, however, chapters 6 through 12 emphasize a more physical approach to pain relief, while chapters 13 through 16 stress psychological aspects. Explore this material with an open mind to select the most promising avenues for pain relief in your own labor.

6

You Are What You Eat:

Nutrition

At no time in your life is good nutrition more crucial than when you are pregnant. Your baby literally depends on you to give him high-quality ingredients for growth. You can ensure your baby's healthy development and your own well-being, too, by eating well while you are pregnant.

In the past, rigid restrictions on maternal weight gain obscured nutrition's important role in contributing to a healthy baby. Thirty years ago mothers were cautioned to gain no more than 15 or 20 pounds. But recent research suggests that the healthiest babies are born to mothers who gain between 25 and 35 pounds. Accordingly, in 1990, the U.S. National Institute of Medicine recommended that most pregnant women should gain this much weight. So instead of counting calories to keep within some predetermined weight limit, pay close attention to eating well.

Getting Ready. Books on nutrition during pregnancy abound. All agree that you need more calories, protein, vitamins, and minerals than you do when you're not pregnant. In the last few weeks of pregnancy, you may not feel as though you have enough room to keep eating well, but try to do so anyway. Your baby grows rapidly and puts on most of his weight during the third trimester. In addition, being well-nourished can help you cope better with the stress of labor.

If you can't handle the traditional pattern of three square meals a day, consider "grazing," that is, eating several smaller meals, and enjoying high-quality snacks—yogurt, nuts, cheese, and fresh fruits and vegetables—between them.

One of the best sources of information on nutrition in pregnancy is a concise pamphlet called *As You Eat, So Your Baby Grows*, by nutritionist Nikki Goldbeck. According to Goldbeck, each day that you're pregnant you should aim to consume:

- One quart of milk (or calcium-containing substitutes like cheese, canned fish with bones, or soybean products).
- Two to four 15-gram servings of high protein foods.
- One serving of dark green leafy vegetables.
- One to two servings of vitamin C-rich foods.
- One yellow or orange vegetable or fruit.
- Four to eight servings of whole grain foods.
- One or two tablespoons of vegetable oil or butter.
- Salt to taste.
- Six to eight glasses of liquid.

It's important, too, to keep taking the vitamin supplement your doctor or midwife recommends. Joanne Slavin, Ph.D., associate professor of nutrition at the University of Minnesota, comments, "It's tough to get all the nutrients you need just from food—iron and folic acid, especially." But beware of high-potency vitamin and mineral supplements during pregnancy. Megadoses of certain vitamins can lead to birth defects, rebound deficiencies, or withdrawal reactions in babies after birth.

Certain vitamins and minerals present in a well-balanced diet and in your vitamin supplement may play a role in easing your labor. In *Let's Have Healthy Children* Adelle Davis recommended a pregnancy diet rich in zinc, potassium, magnesium, and vitamin E to promote an easier and more rapid labor. Because B vitamins are often recommended for stress reduction, a pre-labor diet high in vitamin B-rich foods, such as whole grains, could also aid you in coping with labor's stress.

Unfortunately, books on nutrition for pregnancy drop you off at the hospital door and don't pick you up again until after your baby is born. Why? Because most American women are still cautioned against eating anything during labor. While some women are permitted "labor liquids," many others are forbidden to take anything at all by mouth once active labor has begun. The average first-time mother on this regimen would be going without nourishment for 12 hours. And one in 20 women has a first labor that lasts over 34 hours. Dr. Joanne Slavin says, "If you think of a sporting event as comparable, it's a long time to go without nourishment."

In place of food and drink, most women are given glucose water by an IV, or intravenous line, inserted into the back of the hand. Critics of this regime note that the IV is hardly a food substitute. It doesn't supply a woman with sufficient calories, nor does it assuage the hunger and thirst which normally accompany being without sustenance for many hours while engaging in a strenuous activity.

To Fast or Not To Fast.   Many people—even some doctors—believe that labor stops a woman's digestive system, leaving any food lurking in her stomach as a lethal weapon should she vomit under general anesthesia. Actually, research has shown that unmedicated labor does not stop digestion. Painkillers and lying flat on your back, however, may indeed combine to *slow* the time it takes to digest your food.

In colonial times, American women in labor got hearty food. Tea, toast, buckwheat gruel, mutton, and eggs gave them strength, and red wine cordials promoted relaxation. Later, in his classic obstetrical texts published between 1904 and 1941, Dr. Joseph DeLee maintained that women *should* be given nourishment during labor.

The practice of fasting in labor began only in the 1940s. Fasting, it was thought, would protect women from the aspiration of gastric contents. Aspiration was a grave, often fatal, risk of general anesthesia, which had become prevalent by that time.

According to research on maternal deaths, however, the most important factor in preventing aspiration seems to be not fasting, but rather, the careful administration of anesthesia. Indeed, even fasting cannot provide complete safety under general anesthesia, because a woman might vomit and breathe in gastric acid even from an "empty" stomach.

Since fasting increases the volume and acidity of gastric juices, a pregnant woman administered a general anesthetic should get an antacid "cocktail" prior to receiving anesthesia. To protect women further, a general anesthetic is almost always given by tube, not by mask, in order to prevent the inspiration of foreign matter into a woman's air passage. Under ordinary circumstances, then, eating small amounts of easily digested food in early labor should not pose a grave risk, even if a general anesthetic does become necessary later on.

The controversy is clear: Should women at low risk for the use of a general anesthetic eat and drink to remain comfortable and well-nourished during labor, or should they fast and be supplied with intravenous fluids on the rare chance that they will need general anesthesia and the even more remote possibility that they will suffer an anesthetic accident? Now that general anesthesia is so rarely used in American deliveries, some practitioners believe the practice of routine fasting during labor should be reevaluated.

Doctors and midwives who do home deliveries or births in alternative birthing centers maintain that depriving pregnant women of food and drink for many hours actually puts women at higher risk for longer, more uncomfortable labors. Kathy Dunne, a certified nurse-midwife, says, "If you get a general anesthetic, you shouldn't eat, but hardly anyone gets generals nowadays. You can do a lot more harm by getting hypoglycemic and dehydrated." In fact, hypoglycemia, the lowered blood sugar that comes from fasting, may actually cause the nausea that so many women experience during labor. Laboring women may be like marathon runners, who are apt to become nauseated and vomit if they don't load up on fluids and carbohydrates before a competition.

Dr. Frederic Ettner, a family practitioner who does home deliveries, believes that "a woman in labor absolutely should eat normally before she gets to the hospital." He goes on to caution that "food in labor should be really easy to digest. Women are better off with carbohydrates and very easy-to-digest proteins with carbohydrates, like yogurt. Most of my patients have pieces of fruit, sips of 7-Up, or apple juice."

Light Labor Fare.   If you do eat and drink during labor, what should you have? Available research is sparse; most American women, after all, deliver in hospitals where "nothing by mouth" or "nothing but ice chips" is the rule. But the experiences of attendants who conduct home or home-like births provide some information on what's best to eat in labor.

Certified nurse-midwife Pat Morrow says, "At our alternative birthing center we suggest juices, herb teas, and water—not too many dairy products. We warn them not to go out for pizza or spaghetti if they're in early labor, because that might put them off it for life." Morrow is referring here to the nausea and vomiting that sometimes happen during labor. There are two main periods for this nausea: when a woman first goes into active labor and toward the end of the dilating stage (transition).

In Great Britain, where Morrow received her training, midwives "used to urge large quantities of fluids and we saw much more nausea. Now, we just suggest sips of liquid after each contraction and nausea is less of a problem." A mother recalls, "They brought me juice and encouraged me to drink it. I remember everyone saying 'Keep fluids in your system.'"

Another mother who gave birth at a birthing center in New York recalls going into labor at three in the morning. "The midwives told me I should be drinking juice, not water, as it has no nutritive value. So my husband ran out for some. Thank goodness for the New York City hours! At the 3 A.M. phone call, the midwife also suggested I have a bowl of cereal to give me some strength. She said this might slow down the contractions and give me more blood sugar. As it turned out, I don't think it affected the labor much because the contractions were three to four minutes apart by 6:30 A.M."

Think of yourself as a marathon athlete and plan to eat a "pre-run" meal in early labor. A marathoner would eat a meal high in liquid for hydration; high in carbohydrates such as cereals, bread, or pasta, for quick energy; and low in fat for digestive ease.

Whether or not you feel like eating in early labor, you should certainly keep your fluid intake high. Even a doctor who cautions you against eating in early labor will usually advocate "clear fluids," or fluids you can see through, for nourishment in early labor. Dehydration from being fluid-deprived can actually cause uterine contractions; these usually disappear when you get enough to drink. But sometimes the contractions don't go away. In fact, in Israel, the "Yom Kippur effect" is known to boost the birth rate; observant Jewish women are especially likely to give birth the day after observing the stringent 24-hour fast. You don't want, however, to begin your labor in a dehydrated state.

Depending on your birth attendant's practices and your preference, when you are admitted to the hospital in labor, you'll either be permitted light nourishment—usually clear fluids—or you'll be restricted to a few ice chips or sucks on a popsicle or lollipop.

Again, depending on your individual situation, if you're not permitted to drink, you may have fluids introduced by IV from the beginning of your stay, toward the end, or not at all (see chapter 17). Nurse-midwife Kathy Dunne says, "For most women, oral fluids, not IVs, are the way to go. But if it's a high-risk situation, say prolonged rupture of the membranes, we have to look towards possible intervention and that means an IV."

Taking the Bite out of Labor Pain. No current research indicates that any particular food actually reduces labor pain, but abundant anecdotal lore names several substances that may ease pain or help labor along.

Calcium.   Adelle Davis recommended calcium supplementation, citing its effectiveness in decreasing pain. She wrote, "At the time I was seeing the patients for three obstetricians, I often suggested to these women that they take with a glass of whole milk enough tablets to supply 2000 milligrams of calcium between the time labor started and [the time] they arrived at the hospital. Many had easy deliveries and some declared that they experienced almost no pain." Dr. Joanne Slavin comments, "Calcium lactate is a fairly readily-absorbed form that's useful for muscle cramps. There may be no good controlled studies on it, but there are a lot of anecdotal reports." Nutritionist Nikki Goldbeck concurs that calcium may be helpful in labor: "Some people use it to control cramps; it's not that far-out of an idea." However, she cautions that "calcium can initiate diarrhea in some women."

Vitamin B-complex.   In her book *Birth in Four Cultures*, anthropologist Brigitte Jordan describes the traditional use in the Yucatan of a vitamin B-complex injection as a labor stimulant. Current medical literature lacks information on this use of vitamin B, but Margaret Mead and Niles Newton pointed out the widespread use of vitamin B_1 in Europe during the 1940s and 1950s. They cited research that supported the use of vitamin B_1 both as a labor enhancer and as a pain reliever.

Red raspberry leaf tea.   Dr. Grantly Dick-Read encouraged red raspberry leaf tea as a drink for his laboring patients. Many books on home delivery advocate this brew. You might try taking raspberry leaf tea (available at any health food store) every hour during labor to relieve nausea and promote efficient contractions.

Here's Adelle Davis's recipe: Over one ounce of raspberry leaves (you can buy these at any health food store), pour one pint boiling water. Cover, and let steep for half an hour. Strain the tea, and, as delivery approaches, drink it as hot as possible. If your birth attendant agrees, you could bring the concoction to the hospital in a thermos.

Caulophyllum.   Throughout history, herbal concoctions such as teas, oils, powdered bark, and dried leaves have been employed to promote labor progress or ease labor pain. Homeopathic physicians occasionally recommend caulophyllum, or blue cohosh, during the final week of pregnancy or prescribe it in labor if a woman's contractions are ineffective.

Blue cohosh, however, may be associated with high blood pressure and mucous membrane irritation. Other herbal preparations carry other possible side effects. Nutritionist Nikki Goldbeck cautions, "I'm a little uncomfortable at recommending herbs, a little hesitant to suggest these things for labor." Be sure to consult an herbalist or a homeopathic physician if you intend to use herbal remedies during your labor.

Alcohol. Most pregnant women are so used to doing without alcohol for the good of their babies that they seldom think of it as a means of relaxing in early labor. Alcohol, however, has a long cross-cultural history as a labor pain reliever. In the Ukraine, Ireland, and Guatemala, as well as in colonial America, women were given alcoholic drinks such as whiskey or wine to ease labor pain.

Alcohol does reach the fetus in concentrations similar to those in maternal blood, so it should be considered a drug and used with the same caution. Still, at the end of a full-term pregnancy, you no longer need to be concerned about a glass of wine causing fetal alcohol syndrome. If you are unable to relax by natural means in early labor, you may want to try one-half to one ounce of brandy or whiskey or a small glass of wine. Don't overdo it. As you probably know, too much alcohol can make you quite nauseated. But a minor indulgence in early labor may help to make you feel more relaxed and able to cope.

7

Getting a Buzz On:

Transcutaneous Electrical Nerve Stimulation and Acupuncture

The two methods of pain relief discussed in this chapter—transcutaneous electrical nerve stimulation and acupuncture—both have a long history. Transcutaneous electrical nerve stimulation (TENS), the application of electrical current to the skin, is actually a modern application of an age-old remedy. Records from Roman and Egyptian history describe the use of torpedo fish or electric eels for the relief of migraine and gout. Occasionally the headache disappeared only after the patient had been electrocuted! In its modern guise TENS has proven to be at least as effective as these electrifying methods and much less risky, too.

Acupuncture, on the other hand, hasn't changed all that much since it originated in China over two thousand years ago. The insertion of extremely slender needles into the patient at points seemingly unrelated to his pain or problem, has been an integral feature of Chinese medicine for several millennia. But Western doctors have only recently begun to recognize the usefulness of acupuncture as a legitimate medical aid.

TENS and acupuncture can relieve labor pain as well as some other common problems of pregnancy, and both can promote a more comfortable recovery after delivery (see chapter 20). Because neither therapy comprises part of a typical American doctor's training, you're not likely to hear about TENS or acupuncture from your doctor. But after reading this chapter, you'll be better able to judge whether you'd like to try TENS or acupuncture and you'll have the necessary information to pursue either therapy further.

TENS

Several years ago, Rhonda Kotarinos was called to provide TENS therapy to a woman in labor with her first child. Kotarinos, president of Women's Therapeutic Services in Melrose Park, Illinois, says, "Cindy had been in labor for about 18 hours. After so many hours of pain, she was barely receptive to my suggestions on how to handle the TENS unit. But a year and a half later, when she was pregnant with her second child, she came looking for me. This time she insisted, 'I've got to have that TENS before I go into labor!'"

Kotarinos's client, a dentist named Cindy Jordan-Giannini, says, "I'm a wimp and I don't take pain too well. I don't know how much TENS reduced the contraction pain, but it did allow me to relax between contractions. That was the only thing that kept me from needing medication during both of my labors."

What Is TENS?   TENS applies electrical current to the skin by means of flexible silicone electrodes, placed strategically in pairs and attached to the skin with conducting gel. Small wires connect these electrodes to a pocket-sized, battery-operated stimulator that emits a continuous series of electrical pulses. The patient adjusts the strength of the electrical stimulus and typically reports it to be a comfortable sensation. Russell A. Foley, president of Foley Physical Therapy and Consulting Services in Fayetteville, Georgia, is nationally recognized as a leader in the use of TENS for pain management. Foley says, "TENS is a tingling, tickling, buzzing type of feeling. And people's general response is, 'This feels really good.'"

The gate control theory of Ronald Melzack and Patrick D. Wall best explains how this type of stimulation works to combat pain (see chapter 1). Remember that the sensation of pain frequently travels toward the brain on slow, small, unmyelinated nerve fibers. Electricity from the TENS unit excites fast, large-diameter, myelinated nerve fibers. Because the TENS message travels faster than the pain message, the central nervous system gate closes to pain perception. Researchers generally agree that TENS also stimulates the release of endorphins,

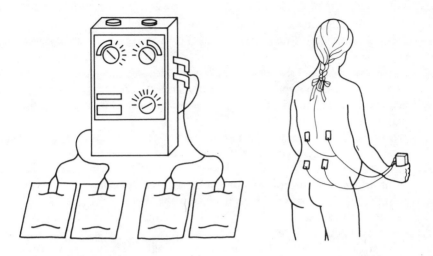

Transcutaneous electrical nerve stimulation (TENS) unit (left), *and the device in use* (right).

the body's naturally-occurring opiates, which further depress pain perception.

First employed in this country for the relief of chronic pain, TENS has recently been used to alleviate postoperative pain, such as post-cesarean pain (see chapter 20). In addition, TENS has been used at acupuncture points to induce contractions in women whose pregnancies have gone past their due dates.

Although TENS is rarely used for labor and delivery in this country, more than a decade of research in Europe has shown that it provides good relief of labor pain with very few drawbacks.

A study by Lars-Erik Augustinnson and his colleagues in Sweden demonstrated that TENS in labor afforded moderate to good pain relief to 130 out of 147 patients. Other studies from Germany and Great Britain concluded that TENS gave good pain relief to about three-quarters of the women who used it during the first stage of labor. A study published in the *British Journal of Obstetrics and Gynaecology* suggested that most of the women using TENS required supplemental medication. Still, the authors concluded that TENS prompted high satisfaction among the women who used it, and that it did not interfere with the signals from the electronic fetal monitor.

Two American studies published in the journal *Physical Therapy* found that TENS offered at least moderate pain relief to four out of five of the women who tried it. While most American hospitals do not offer TENS as a standard form of pain relief in labor, physical therapy personnel know how to use TENS and can assist obstetric patients in its use.

In labor, TENS electrodes typically get placed in two pairs on either side of the woman's spine. One pair of electrodes, for first stage labor, goes near her waist. The other pair, for second stage labor, goes at the very base of her spine.

Since this placement of electrodes does not alleviate pain in the groin, some writers advocate placing electrodes on the abdomen or groin during late first stage and second stage labor. So far, this placement has caused no problems for mothers or babies. Other practitioners recommend putting the electrodes on the woman's thighs or even her ankles because these points are far from the baby and the ankle point is an acupuncture point.

Though TENS does afford excellent pain relief to some women, it is not a panacea for labor pain. A small percentage of women get no relief from TENS at all.

Most women describe TENS as giving moderate to good pain relief, and they usually use it as an adjunct to the breathing and relaxing methods learned in childbirth class. You should consider TENS as a sort of "super massage" rather than as an anesthetic that will completely remove your labor pain.

Is TENS Safe?   Conventional—that is to say, chemical—methods for labor pain relief all carry some degree of risk to mother and baby (see chapter 18). Thus far, TENS appears to be free of any negative effect on either mother or baby. Rhonda Kotarinos says, "When mothers use TENS, babies' Apgar scores are equal to or better than those of women who took nothing. Unlike drugs, TENS can be turned off any time during labor and its effects don't linger. It doesn't lower a mother's blood pressure or give her nausea the way a shot of Demerol might. And you don't have the increased risk of a cesarean or a forceps delivery that you get with the epidural."

Critics caution that the use of TENS in labor may have unknown negative effects on infants. Because the baby is a bioelectric system and is surrounded by water, which conducts electricity, the use of TENS in labor is still considered experimental. In addition, some critics claim that a woman using TENS can quickly become habituated to the electrical stimulus, which would radically decrease its effectiveness in a short time.

You can avoid habituation by changing the parameters of the stimulation. Russell Foley comments, "There are three main controls you can work with—the amplitude, the duration, and the frequency of the stimulus. You can also reverse the lead wires. And so, by changing all these different parameters, you can reduce the adaptation factor. In addition, as each contraction starts to build, you can set it so that the amplitude is automatically boosted. And after the contraction peaks and descends, the toggle switch can be flipped back to the baseline, thereby lowering the stimulus."

TENS in Your Hospital. The biggest obstacle to your use of TENS in labor will probably be your doctor's reluctance to try something new when he or she already has confidence in the more familiar chemical methods for pain relief. TENS is not something you can go out and buy for your own use; as a prescription product, it's available by physician referral only. Furthermore, you'll need some orientation, preferably before labor, to get the most out of the use of TENS. You need to learn how to set it up, where to put the electrodes, and how and when to adjust the parameters of stimulation.

In the handful of hospitals where TENS is regularly used for labor and delivery, you would come in to the physical therapy department about four weeks before your due date. A physical therapist would explain the use of the TENS instrument to you. You'd put it on and experiment with different magnitudes of stimulation, to learn how to control the rate of electrical impulses and to increase their intensity when needed.

If your hospital doesn't use TENS routinely for labor and delivery—and most don't—you'll have to get a special prescription from your doctor to use it for your labor. You may run into opposition. Russell Foley cautions, "Classically, the OB/GYN hasn't been involved in physical therapy. This is a new area for him. Since he hasn't been using it and he doesn't have colleagues using it, he's hesitant to try something new in his field. Now, family practitioners who have patients with sports injuries or chronic back pain have used TENS, and they may show less hesitation because they've used it in a different patient population and achieved success. But until there's more documentation in this country, there's going to be some hesitation on the part of most doctors to use TENS in obstetrics."

You might try calling your hospital's physical therapy department for information. Let your doctor know that research indicates TENS does not interfere with fetal monitoring and has no proven ill effects on the baby.

If you plan to have your baby in a hospital whose physical therapy department uses TENS—and almost all of them do—your doctor could write a prescription for you to go to the department to learn how to use the unit. TENS units can be rented on a monthly basis with your doctor's prescription and most insurance companies will reimburse you for the rental expense. Be sure to look into this with your own insurance company, though, because the rental fee may exceed $75 or $100 per month.

If you plan to use TENS in labor, you'll be in charge of how much stimulation you receive. Late in the first stage, however, some women like to let their labor partner or nurse take over adjusting the controls. Some critics argue that TENS just uses pain to counteract pain, but advocates claim that women in labor are helped by their use of TENS. Russell Foley says, "A lot of times when you first put them on TENS, there's a great sigh of relief and the women say, 'It feels like my husband's massaging my back.' The husband's sitting in the corner with his poor hands all fatigued and he looks really happy too!"

Acupuncture

Used in China for at least 2,000 years, acupuncture first came to mainstream attention in the United States in 1971. When *New York Times* writer James Reston had an emergency appendectomy while traveling in China, acupuncture needles relieved his postoperative abdominal discomfort. After Reston wrote about his experience, some American doctors went to China to learn acupuncture. Since then, schools of acupuncture have been established in several states. According to the American Association for Acupuncture and Oriental Medicine (AAAOM), approximately 5,000 acupuncturists currently practice in the United States and 300 new ones get certified each year.

Some Americans have seen the documentary film of a young Chinese woman having a cesarean delivery under acupuncture anesthesia and calmly eating an apple immediately after surgery. Even in China, however, acupuncture was not used as a surgical anesthetic until 1958; today it's used this way only about 20 percent of the time, and it is frequently supplemented by tranquilizers. In the United States, acupuncture is rarely used as an anesthetic at all.

But even if acupuncture's anesthetic applications are limited, many American doctors have come to accept it as an extremely effective treatment for some types of chronic pain; for disorders like ulcers, colitis, hypertension, asthma, allergies, and premenstrual syndrome; and for treating a variety of sports injuries. In some cases, acupuncture may be a useful therapy for a pregnant woman. According to Pam Mills, a board-certified acupuncturist in Chicago, pregnancy and birth problems that can often be relieved with acupuncture include morning sickness, malposition of the fetus, prolonged labor, retained placenta, postnatal spasm and pain, and insufficient milk. "Acupuncture," says Mills, "is a viable alternative to Western medicine, one with a tremendous history."

How Does Acupuncture Work? According to Chinese theory, the body's vital energy, *qi* (pronounced chee), travels through the body along twelve major pathways called meridians. Each of the six meridians on the legs and each of the six on the arms connects with a major organ. When the patient's *qi* is disrupted by inner or outer forces, acupuncturists redirect this energy by needling particular points along the meridians. These points are the acupuncture points. Manipulating the *qi* in this fashion achieves a proper balance of *yin* (the feminine life force) with *yang* (the masculine life force). Keeping a balance between *yin* and *yang*, acupuncturists say, forms the basis of psychological and physical health.

Acupuncture does not exist as an isolated therapy—if you have such-and-such a problem, treat it with such-and-such a needle—but rather forms part of a complex and metaphorical worldview in which health is considered more than simply the absence of a verifiable disease. In contrast to Western medicine, which analyzes test results to find the cause of an illness and treat it, Chinese medicine is more concerned with manipulating a pattern of disharmony in order to restore health by activating the body's own mechanisms for healing.

Thus Chinese medicine does not differentiate between psychological and physiological causes of illness, but rather assesses the whole system to arrive at a diagnosis which will treat the person's body and mind. Acupuncturist Mills says, "I get people who say, 'My doctor insists nothing is wrong just because it wasn't on the test.' All the tests Western doctors do are really important, but you have to look at people in terms of their faces, how they're sitting, how they act."

Western scientists looking at acupuncture have been at somewhat of a loss in trying to explain how it works in a way that makes sense to the Western mind. Traditional acupuncture points appear to an unschooled observer to have absolutely nothing to do with the problems being treated. But according to a recent editorial in the *British Medical Journal*, "If acupuncture provides effective and safe pain relief, then its mechanism of action is of secondary importance." In other words, if it works, it doesn't matter how.

Some experts believe that acupuncture activates the body's own system of naturally occurring painkillers—not only the endorphins, but also the related enkephalins as well as serotonin, another neurotransmitter associated with pain relief.

However acupuncture works, it has thousands of years of experience behind it. Despite the American Medical Association's classification of acupuncture as "experimental," one American doctor who uses acupuncture in his psychiatric practice says, "It's Western medicine—only 50 years old—that should be considered the experiment!"

Would You Benefit from Acupuncture?   In an article on acupuncture in pregnancy for *Mothering,* acupuncturist Mobi Ho described several benefits of acupuncture for pregnant women. For example, Ho recommended consulting with an acupuncturist if you are bothered by morning sickness that does not respond to changes in your diet. She wrote, "Chinese medicine does not look on morning sickness as simply a natural, inevitable part of pregnancy. . . . Rather, it is an imbalance which pregnancy has either caused or exacerbated by placing stress on what may already be a delicate balance in the woman's health."

Needles aren't always necessary in the Chinese treatment of morning sickness. Ho wrote that some women find relief by applying pressure at the acupuncture points associated with this problem: "One can palpate for tender spots 2–3 inches up from the wrist on the inside of the arm between the two large tendons for points. Apply deep pressure at these points with your thumb for several seconds at times throughout the day."

Acupuncture may also be helpful during pregnancy to turn a breech (bottom-first) fetus to a vertex or head-first position. Scientific papers from China say that breech babies can be turned safely and effectively by means of an acupuncture technique called moxibustion—that is, the burning of the herb moxa (a specially aged mugwort) near the lower outside corner of the mother's little toenail, an acupuncture point. A fetus whose mother is treated by this technique, the papers claim, turns himself to the correct position 90 percent of the time compared to only 60 percent for untreated mothers. Since most American doctors routinely deliver breech babies by cesarean section, this treatment might help you avoid unnecessary surgery (see chapter 17). Pam Mills comments, "I would treat a woman for a malpositioned fetus, but first I would make sure she had been checked out by a doctor to confirm that there was no reason the baby could not safely be repositioned."

Acupuncture may also be used to prevent premature labor, or, conversely, to induce postmature labor. In the Chinese literature, acupuncture induction has proven as effective as induction by Pitocin, while being associated with fewer side effects to the mother and fetus. TENS stimulation at acupuncture points may also prove effective in inducing labor.

Unless your obstetrician, family practitioner, or midwife is trained in acupuncture, it's unlikely that you'll be offered the option of using this method to alleviate labor pain. But if you've been treated by an acupuncturist during pregnancy, your practitioner may be permitted to accompany you to the hospital in labor. Be sure to pave the way for this arrangement with your own birth attendant well in advance of your labor.

If you can't arrange to have acupuncture during labor, ask your acupuncturist to place small stimulation beads on your ears or other body parts in early labor. Sharon Feng, an acupuncturist with 23 years of experience at the Shanghai Second Medical College of Obstetrics and Gynecology, currently practices at Five Branches Traditional Chinese Medical Clinic in Santa Cruz, California. Feng says, "With these beads, self-massage or an assistant's massage may be more helpful than simple massage without the beads. It's less ideal than complete acupuncture treatment, but can be an excellent help under the circumstances."

Experienced acupuncturists stress that acupuncture points may be massaged or pressed rather than needled, and that acupressure is something you can do yourself to help your labor progress more efficiently. We'll describe acupressure points for labor and how to massage them in chapter 8.

Selecting an Acupuncturist.   If you decide you'd like to explore this avenue for promoting a healthier pregnancy and a more efficient labor, you might begin your search by calling or writing the American Association for Acupuncture and Oriental Medicine (see Resources). AAAOM can let you know how your state regulates the practice of acupuncture and can tell you if a particular practitioner has passed a qualifying exam given by the National Commission for the Certification of Acupuncturists. Or, you could call your state or local medical society. According to a recent article in *Time* magazine, acupuncture is illegal in 24 states unless it's practiced by a medical doctor. But more than 20 other states license, certify, or register nonphysician acupuncturists who have passed the national exam.

An article on acupuncture for *East West Journal* states that "finding a good acupuncturist is about as important as finding a good auto mechanic and as difficult as finding a good spouse." Here are some suggestions for finding an acupuncturist.

After soliciting referrals from your doctor, from a local pain clinic, from AAAOM, or from friends who have used an acupuncturist, arrange for a consultation. Many practitioners offer a free consultation; once there, you should ask to see a diploma from a reputable school of acupuncture.

The first exam should take about an hour and a half. You'll be asked a lot of questions about your history, symptoms, diet, and any prior treatments. Your skin and tongue will be examined and you'll have your pulse read at several different points (the tongue and pulses are important diagnostic tools in this system). A good acupuncturist should explain everything and suggest diet and lifestyle changes, not just a course of needle therapy. Generally, the practitioner will be able to predict about how many treatments you will need, and he or she should not make incredible claims for miracle cures.

If you sign on for a treatment, you'll usually receive needles in your forearms, hands, legs, or feet—occasionally in your trunk—depending on the acupuncturist's assessment of your situation. You will get six to thirty needles. Their lengths will vary, but they will all be extremely thin.

You can hardly feel the needles except for a very slight tingle. They're left in place for a few minutes to over an hour, during which time the acupuncturist may leave them alone or may gently twirl them. During the treatment, the practitioner should reexamine your pulses to see if your energy is coming back into balance; this would signal an end to the treatment.

Sometimes, as described above, moxibustion rather than acupuncture will be selected as the proper mode of treatment—for a fetal repositioning from breech position, for example.

Despite the strangeness of having needles put into unexpected places in your body, acupuncture involves no known risk. Bleeding is extremely rare and the thin stainless steel needles, half an inch to four inches long, are sterilized between uses. The main risk is not improper placement of the needles, but rather the possible failure to recognize an underlying disease which requires treatment with Western medicine. That's why it's essential to have your doctor check you thoroughly before going to an acupuncturist in pregnancy.

Depending on your insurance company, you may or may not receive reimbursement for acupuncture treatment. Check your own policy to see if your company requires a doctor's prescription to reimburse you partially or fully for treatment. Charges vary greatly from place to place, but they tend to be higher where insurance companies reimburse for acupuncture treatment. Call around to compare fees. Some acupuncturists apply a sliding scale, depending on your ability to pay. Acupuncture costs can vary between $20 and $60 per treatment, so it's important to learn how many treatments will be necessary and at what cost before embarking upon a course of acupuncture.

8
Rubbing Where It Hurts:
Massage, Counterpressure, and Acupressure

What do you do when you're in pain? If you're like most people, you probably massage or stroke the painful part of your body. Or, you may simply apply stationary pressure, or *counterpressure*. It's an instinctive reaction to touch yourself where it hurts. And being stroked by someone else can often afford you even greater relief.

Massage and manipulation techniques for pain appear in history's most ancient medical records. The oldest medical work in existence—an Egyptian document dating from 1550 B.C.—included prescriptions for massage with various oils and herbs. Hippocrates himself asserted that anyone who aspired to be a physician had first to master the art of massage.

You don't have to understand anything about how massage works to appreciate being touched in a relieving way. But the more you know, the better you can put this powerful technique to work for you during pregnancy and labor.

Massage in Pregnancy

Massage offers several benefits during pregnancy. Kathy Cain, a registered massage therapist and author of *Partners in Birth,* says, "Massage gets pregnant women comfortable with and aware of their own bodies. It creates a relaxed atmosphere for the person and is a nurturing, caring kind of experience—something pregnant women and new mothers both really need. If a pregnant woman's partner massages her, this experience can literally get the couple in touch with one another."

Kathy Cain spoke as she massaged Celeste Roy, then eight months pregnant with her first child. As Cain began the luxurious massage, aided by many strategically placed pillows, lovely mood music, and scented oil, she remarked, "Normally, we'd not be talking at all; I'd encourage Celeste to get into her breathing, just relaxing as she exhales."

Cain gave extra attention to Celeste's trouble spots, saying, "Not just Celeste, but most of us hold lots of tension in the upper back and shoulders. When I massage them, women say, 'Oh, you've found it.' But it's no big secret. In labor, a woman's partner could easily massage her shoulders and shoulder blades from behind if the woman were straddling a chair, lying on her side, or kneeling in the labor bed."

The 45-minute massage was a success for Celeste Roy, in spite of the fact that Kathy Cain's commentary competed with the music: "I feel so relaxed," said Celeste, stretching languorously. "Yes," said Cain. "And hopefully, you'll feel more alive and energetic too."

A good massage can leave you feeling energized and relaxed at the same time, because the process of being stroked and rubbed releases muscle tension. If tension is a problem for you, massage may be just the key you need to help you relax.

A professional massage during pregnancy can be a wonderful treat. According to James Hackett, co-director of the Chicago School of Massage Therapy, an hour of professional massage typically costs between $40 and $60.

First, find out what kind of training a massage therapist has had. The American Massage Therapy Association (AMTA) boasted 12,000 members in 1991 and provides a national referral service (see Resources). AMTA's Council of Schools oversees 60 certified massage schools around the country where practitioners receive a standardized training program including a minimum of 500 hours of instruction. Ask if your practitioner has been certified by AMTA. "You should also ask what kind of experience this person has in working with pregnant women," suggests Hackett. "This training is available and we do address it in our program."

Even if you decide to make massage strictly a do-it-yourselves project, you can still reap tremendous benefits from the activity. Hackett suggests taking a class at a local massage school or outreach program. "Often, there are workshops specific to massage for couples. These can teach you how to do some basic things. You'll get the relaxing effects of massage, some nurturing, and a nice bond between you and your husband."

If your partner is interested, he can learn some useful techniques from a massage demonstration, or simply by trying it and responding sensitively to your reactions.

In his introduction to *Massage and Peaceful Pregnancy*, Gordon Inkeles writes that massage is something special a husband can do to help his wife on a daily basis throughout pregnancy. Addressing his remarks to expectant fathers, Inkeles says, "She can *feel* that you care because during a massage nothing is more important to you than her well-being."

Inkeles suggests the following necessities for a good massage: a firm, warm surface for the woman to lie on; plenty of pillows for positioning her limbs and keeping her back straight; a light, clear vegetable oil (like coconut or almond) kept in a small plastic squeeze bottle to prevent spills; and towels. Music, candlelight, incense, and fragrance to scent the oil are extras—lovely, but not strictly necessary.

Here are the do's and don'ts of massage:

Do:

- Keep your fingers together when you knead and stroke.
- Maintain constant physical contact with your partner.
- Make your movements rhythmic and smooth.
- Keep the room warm.
- Use just enough oil to ease your strokes.
- Attend to your partner's likes and dislikes.
- Pay attention to all parts of your partner's body.
- Adjust the pillows for her comfort.

Don't:

- Bear down too hard near where she feels pain.
- Talk too much.
- Watch the clock.
- Allow her to get cold or uncomfortable.
- Do anything that hurts her.
- Massage against a doctor's advice or if your partner is ill.

■ Massage too close to a bruise, cut, inflamed joint, blood clot, tumor, or sensitive veins.

You may want to try again the touch relaxation techniques described on page 60, but this time, have your husband stroke you without telling you to tense up first. He should linger as long as you want on your particular areas for holding tension—your neck and shoulders, perhaps, or maybe your back. His hands, of course, should be warm and relaxed.

In late pregnancy, you shouldn't lie flat on your back to be massaged, so get massaged as you lie first on one side; then, with help, turn onto the other side. If you position the pillows just right, or if you have a special massage or pregnancy pillow (see Resources), you can even get comfortable on your belly. Put regular pillows under your breasts and hips so that your back doesn't sag in the middle. All your limbs should be supported and slightly bent, resting on top of the pillows.

There's almost no part of your body that can't be massaged pleasurably. "Squeeze her feet," Kathy Cain advises labor partners. "You just push in with your fist on the bottom of her foot and then squeeze the top of her foot with your other hand. It takes no skill and it feels wonderful during labor. The buttocks, too, feel great when they're rubbed or kneaded. That's a huge muscle and it's rarely touched."

You might also appreciate receiving a thorough head massage during pregnancy. Later, when you are in labor, your partner can help you relax between pushing contractions from his position behind your head in the delivery room. Your partner can follow these instructions to give a head massage:

> Stroke down the sides of her forehead and at her temples. (Firm pressure with one hand on top of the other at her forehead can ease the pain of a headache.)
> Lift and stroke around her chin and jaw and use very light pressure with your fingertips around her eyes.
> Gently pull her hair up and massage her scalp.
> Trace around the backs of her ears and pinch her earlobes between your fingers.
> Take your time, and repeat the strokes she especially likes.

Pregnancy is often accompanied by an aching back that makes a good back rub more a necessity than a luxury. A complete back massage for the pregnant woman is a fine idea as long as her back pain isn't intense and she has no associated shooting pains down her legs. Back massage triples the blood supply to the woman's muscles, and, as Gordon Inkeles writes, will "leave your partner smiling whether she's hurting or not." Always stroke along the sides of the spine, not the center. If a spot is particularly painful, anchor yourself with one hand as you circle slowly and as deeply as she likes with the palm or heel of your other hand.

Practice the massage techniques you'll most likely be using during labor: stroking, kneading, and pressure. Stroking and kneading require oil (cream absorbs too quickly into the skin), while pressure strokes should be done dry to maximize the effect of the friction. Stroke and knead with the hands open and the fingers together. Kneading, a simple squeezing and release, feels especially good on large muscle areas like the buttocks and thighs. Deep pressure can be applied with the knuckles, the heel of the hand or foot, the forearm, or the tips of the fingers or thumbs. Pressure works well to alleviate pain in a specific location because it's numbing and it decreases circulation to the affected area. During labor, if the masseur's hand should tire, he can wrap it in a soft T-shirt or replace it for a while with a can of tennis balls or another suitable firm item. Technique is probably less important here than endurance.

This may surprise you both, but it's perfectly permissible to massage a pregnant woman's abdomen as long as you avoid any deep pressure. Cup your hands to fit the curve of your partner's belly and give your wife *and* baby a massage.

Even if you've just massaged your wife's back and abdomen, or perhaps just her head and her feet, give her a full body sweep to leave her with the feeling that all of her body has been attended to. As she lies on her side, begin with your two hands at her hip. Move one hand up her body and one hand down her body, then return to her hip with the same amount of pressure. Repeat several times.

Feel free to improvise, always remembering the basic do's and don'ts of massage and being sensitive to your wife's signals that she likes or doesn't like what you're doing. Don't ever hesitate to linger on something she particularly enjoys.

Perineal Massage.   Recent research suggests that perineal massage may decrease the need for an episiotomy (see chapter 17) and the likelihood of a tear. So you may want to oil and massage your perineum each day after your bath. Because perineal massage prepares your skin to stretch more easily when the baby is born, this prior preparation may help keep you from tensing up when your perineum begins to sting shortly before your baby is born. You may want to try perineal massage daily for about five minutes, starting four to six weeks before your due date. But don't do perineal massage if you have herpes or a vaginal infection.

Sit in a comfortable position. Using oil or a water-soluble jelly (not baby oil, mineral oil, or Vaseline), allow your thumbs (or your partner's index fingers) to describe a U-shaped or sling movement around the bottom portion of your vagina. Rub the skin between your thumbs and index fingers, giving yourself just enough pressure so that you feel a stinging sensation. Focus on releasing as you feel the pressure.

Massage and Counterpressure During Labor

Touch can be a tremendous help during labor. The application of very firm pressure relieves pain. Long strokes and kneading promote general relaxation and increase circulation to chilled extremities.

Massage is not only a boon to the mother, however. Massaging a laboring mother can benefit her baby as well. In *Touching*, Ashley Montagu maintained that women who were touched during labor and delivery used their own hands more effectively to caress their babies after birth. Montagu wrote that it would be a good idea to "institute the practice of regular body caressing by the husband of his wife during pregnancy, labor, and after the birth of the baby."

Each woman is different, though. Some love to be massaged during labor while others have been known to yell, "Don't touch me!" when their contractions get intense. A husband doesn't have to take this as a blanket prohibition, however. "If she yells 'don't touch me,' you should ask 'where?'" advises Suzanna May Hilbers, a physical therapist and former faculty member for ASPO/Lamaze. "Light touch may be painful to her while deep touch—hugging, squeezing, or firm counterpressure—could be just the thing she needs."

Under stress some people interpret light touch as potentially dangerous, while firm pressure can feel comforting. Since light touch travels along the same nerve fibers as pain—the free nerve endings, associated with the hair follicles—a light feathery touch may actually worsen pain rather than relieve it.

For some women, the effleurage (fingertip massage of the abdomen) traditionally taught in Lamaze class is irritating, not relaxing. It can be especially irritating if you lightly stroke your abdomen *against* the direction of your hair growth. If you'd like to do effleurage, try it *with* the direction of hair growth and with moderate pressure rather than a light fingertip touch. One mother says, "The pressure of massaging my stomach helped relieve the pain of the contractions and helped me regain control."

Fortunately, other types of touch and pressure sensation race to the brain more quickly than does either pain or light touch. The sensory nerve endings that transmit these sensations to your brain are called Meissner's Corpuscles, Merkel's Disks, and Pacinian Corpuscles.

Meissner's Corpuscles respond to touch. Located in all parts of the skin without hair, they predominate in the fingertips, lips, and feet. The brain is particularly dense with receptors for messages from these areas, especially the fingertips. Try such pain-racing strategies as holding your partner's hand, or stroking something that feels good to you—for example, rose petals or velvet. Many women apply lipstick or gloss between contractions, thereby stimulating their lips and fingertips at the same time. Or you could kiss your husband or give him a mini-massage. A mother recalls, "In order to keep relaxed, I rubbed my hands together or effleuraged Stan's belly."

Merkel's Disks are found in hairy and hairless areas. They respond to continuous deep touch, such as cuddling or being held firmly. Many women appreciate having their husbands cradle them or grip their thighs firmly, even though they might be extremely irritable at a light, ticklish touch. Water, which we'll be discussing in chapter 9, affords a particularly effective means of surrounding yourself with continuous touch.

The Pacinian Corpuscles, especially abundant in hairless zones like your palms and the soles of your feet, respond to deep pressure and vibration. That's why a hand or foot massage can feel wonderful during labor. You might also try a vibrating pillow to stimulate these nerve endings. You can lean on this pillow during labor and use it later to calm a crying baby.

Stimulating any of these three kinds of fast-moving nerve fibers works to reduce pain by closing your central nervous system gate to the slower-moving fibers that conduct pain (see chapter 1). Massage or counterpressure techniques also alleviate pain by making you more relaxed in general.

Where should your partner massage you during labor? The back of the neck and the shoulders frequently hold tension which can spread to the rest of your body. He could also try a firm foot or hand massage, or a lighter massage on your abdomen. A sensitive partner should know if you have particular problem areas, and stroke or knead these during your labor.

The most popular spot for massage in labor is the low back. Here are some methods for doing this type of massage:

- Try firm pressure with your thumbs on either side of her spine. When you get to the right spot, apply pressure or vibrate your thumbs if she finds that this feels good.

■ With the flat of your palm or the heel of your hand, make slow, rhythmic circles around her sacrum (the lowest part of the back).

■ Anchoring yourself with one hand on her hip, put the heel of your palm on her coccyx (tailbone) and cup your hand around her bottom, allowing her low back to feel the warmth of your fingers.

■ Apply firm counterpressure where she needs it with your fist, heel, palm, forearm, or by sitting back to back with her.

You should know that touch techniques may lose their effectiveness after 20 or 30 minutes. If your back pain recurs or worsens, try alternating these methods with heat or cold (see chapter 9), which stimulate other nerve fibers and can give the pressure-sensitive fibers a temporary respite.

Each woman will like a different technique, so experiment until you find what works best for you. One mother said, "The flat of John's hand on my back—rotating hard, but not too hard—felt the best." Another mother appreciated firm pressure, but without rotation. She commented, "The only way I could tolerate the contractions was to have Steve apply steady pressure to my lower back. I found it worked well if he increased the pressure as the monitor showed the contractions getting stronger. He tried massaging my lower back but I couldn't tolerate that. I just loved his warm hands applying pressure during the contractions."

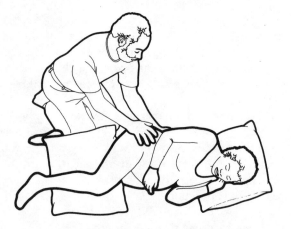

In one type of back massage for labor, you assume a side-lying position in bed or on the floor, with a pillow between your knees. Your partner anchors himself with one hand on your hip.

When James Hackett accompanied one of his school's graduates to the hospital during her labor, he discovered another method for alleviating back labor. "When Cynthia started feeling a lot of lower back pain, I began compressing down into the top of her pelvis and into her gluteal muscles," reports Hackett. (The gluteal muscles are the large muscles of the buttocks.) "She was curled on her side and I was facing her back toward her feet. I leaned with my weight and applied steady, firm pressure on her gluteus. I think some of the actual effect was stretching her lower back. As long as I did this, it took away a lot of the pain of the contractions. Between contractions, I did some more general compression, leaning down and working the muscles of her back with a circular palm motion.

"Even with fetal monitoring I could still massage her back. As she pushed, I massaged her legs, using techniques to relieve cramps in her calves. With labor," continues Hackett, "the need for massage is greater and different than it is during pregnancy. You need directness and deeper pressure. To encourage the woman to relax her body, you have to match the intensity of what's going on in labor."

Acupressure or Shiatsu

Shiatsu, from the Japanese *shi* for finger and *atsu* for pressure, is based on the theory of acupuncture (see chapter 7). Acupuncture without needles, or *acupressure* as it is sometimes called, can be performed by your partner to help your labor progress more efficiently and comfortably.

Four main *tsubos* or pressure points have been associated with the enhancement of labor and the provision of pain relief. *Because pressure on these points strengthens contractions, don't manipulate them before your due date*, unless, for example, an experienced acupuncturist is attempting to rotate your baby to a more advantageous position for birth. Take care, also, not to apply pressure or heat to an area of infection; to red, broken or swollen skin; or to major blood vessels.

You can tell when you've located an acupressure point because these points are extremely sensitive to firm pressure. You can feel a sort of "buzzing" when you press it. The acupressure points that can help labor are Spleen 6, Large Intestine 4, Bladder 67, and Bladder 60.

Locate Spleen 6 by measuring three inches or the width of four fingers upward from the top of your anklebone on the inside of your leg. Slide off the shinbone toward the back of your leg; your partner can press hard here with his thumb, inward toward your shinbone, to relieve your labor pain and speed labor along.

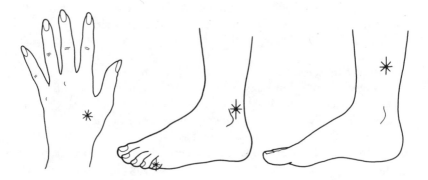

Acupressure points. Left, the Ho-ku *point (Large Intestine 4). Center, Bladder 60, behind the ankle, and Bladder 67, near little toe. Right, Spleen 6.*

Large Intestine 4, also known as the *Ho-ku* point, has been termed a panacea point because it's said to promote overall well-being. Find this point on the back of each hand in the webbing between the thumb and the index finger, about one inch in from the edge of the webbing. With his thumb, your partner can press here, pushing toward your forefinger. Research has shown that simultaneously stimulating Spleen 6 and Large Intestine 4 can induce labor.

Bladder 67 is one tenth of an inch to the outside of the bottom corner of your little toenail. Your husband uses a vibrating sort of pressure with his thumbnail here; pressing this point intensely can help to block painful sensation in your pelvis, affording you some relief from your contractions.

You can find Bladder 60 on the outside of your foot in the depression just to the back of your ankle, midway between the knob of your anklebone and your Achilles tendon. According to *The Path of Pregnancy*, by Bob Flaws, this is "a very useful and efficient point to use for pain control during labor. Finger pressure is usually sufficient, although considerable pressure may have to be applied."

If your partner can do it, it's best to apply hard pressure at the points behind both ankles simultaneously for up to a minute at a time. He may prefer to apply the pressure three times for 10 to 15 seconds at a time, resting a few seconds in between each burst, and repeating every few minutes. If you like it, he can massage the points with a small circular movement, about two to three cycles per second. Your partner should maintain his own comfort by sitting when possible, or by keeping bent knees and a straight back while standing.

9

Some Like It Hot and Some Like It Cold:
Water

Like Robert Frost, who pondered the relative merits of fire and ice, the medical profession has at various times recommended heat or cold as the best method of relieving pain. Actually, both heat and cold can reduce muscle spasms and increase your pain threshold. Depending on your preference, you may use either or both during labor.

Heat dilates blood vessels and speeds the removal of the painful by-products of muscle work. Because heat excels at relieving tension and promoting overall relaxation, it is usually recommended for low-to-moderate levels of pain.

Cold can numb a painful area, constrict blood vessels, and slow the transmission of pain impulses along nerve pathways. Because cold penetrates two to three times more deeply than does heat, and cold receptors in the brain far outnumber heat receptors, it's often recommended for acute discomfort.

Some Like It Hot. When you're feeling achy and sore, you probably head for a warm shower or bath. In early labor, a good long soak will probably relax you in the same way. Most doctors recommend that you stay out of the tub if you think your water has broken. They fear that water with bacteria may enter your vagina, increasing the likelihood of infection. Other practitioners believe that it's safe to take a bath in your own clean tub because it contains household bacteria to which you are already resistant. In fact, a Danish study revealed no increased infection in women who bathed throughout labor. A warm shower is perfectly all right regardless of the condition of your membranes.

One mother says, "Mike called the doctor, had breakfast, and finished packing the Lamaze bag while I took a long shower. I figured I might not get to take one for a while. So there I was taking a shower during what turned out to be late active labor. But it really relieved my back pain."

As many hospital rooms now do, your hospital may boast a shower, hot tub, or even a Jacuzzi for you to use after you've been admitted in labor. Boston's Beth Israel Hospital, for example, has both a shower room and a tub room with a Jacuzzi. Rebecca Rosen-Horn, a childbirth educator and former labor and delivery nurse at Beth Israel, says, "I tell my students the bath or the shower is the place to go when you're not going anywhere in your labor."

Check with your doctor about what facilities are available at your own birthing place. If you'd like, you can even pack a bathing suit for your labor partner.

A mother who used the shower in her hospital's birthing room says, "We were in there about three-quarters of an hour. I sat or stood in the shower and Don used the shower massage on my lower back and abdomen. It felt wonderful!"

Dr. Michel Odent became famous for using a warm water pool at his clinic in Pithiviers, France, to help women relax in labor. Odent wrote that water gave a laboring woman these benefits:

- Water reduces a woman's inhibitions toward giving birth by diminishing catecholamines, the stress hormones.
- Water allows women to enter a different, more primitive level of consciousness.
- Water promotes relaxation, especially if the room is semi-dark and sounds are reduced.
- Water makes contractions more efficient and less painful, thereby shortening labor.

Soaking in warm water during labor can be invaluable for a woman with painful contractions, especially if she's experiencing back labor. In this situation, labor often stalls at around five centimeters. That's the time when many women take painkilling drugs. Dr. Odent observed that if a woman waits to get into the pool until she is five-centimeters dilated, her cervix often dilates completely within about one or two hours after she gets into the water.

Occasionally a shower is sufficient to gain these benefits, particularly if it affords a woman the privacy Odent believes is essential to the laboring process. In his recent book, *Water and Sexuality*, Dr. Odent writes, "A shower in a small private room can be more effective than a bath in a large busy one." Once in a while the mere sight of the pool filling up releases a woman's inhibitions so much that her baby decides to come before she even gets a chance to climb into the pool! And some babies decide to come while their mothers are still reclining in the pool.

After 100 babies accidentally had been born under water at Pithiviers, Odent published his findings in the medical journal *Lancet.* Only two of the 100 babies born in the pool needed any suctioning or help with beginning to breathe. There were no episiotomies and only 29 first-degree (superficial) lacerations, no infections even when the mother's amniotic sac had been broken, and no deaths. Odent concluded that underwater birth did not seem to pose any serious risks for the healthy mother or her baby.

At the Family Birthing Center in Upland, California, 483 women purposely gave birth in water, between February 1985 and June 1989. Babies all emerged with good Apgar scores and only one mother suffered a minor infection. Dr. Michael Rosenthal, who has assisted in almost 800 water births at the center, commented on doctors' and mothers' different reactions at first view of the center's pool: "Pregnant women rarely ask why one would use a bath in labor; physicians usually do."

Some American mothers actively seek out underwater birth for their babies; in this type of birth, the mother rests in a tub of water heated to around 100 degrees and the baby stays submerged for several minutes after birth. Adherents of underwater birth say it reduces birth stress and unnecessary interventions for both mother and baby. Opponents of underwater birth fear that the baby will get an infection or that water will enter his bloodstream. Even advocates of underwater birth caution that the newborn's vital signs, umbilical cord, and placenta must be examined scrupulously to avoid serious problems. (See the Resources section of this book for information on ordering or building a portable birthing tub.)

If your birthing place doesn't boast a hot tub or shower for relaxing in labor, you may find it helpful just to soak your hands or feet in a basin of warm water. Your labor partner could warm some lotion or oil in hot water and give you a backrub. Or try using a hot water bottle, heating pad, or hot compresses where you need them most: on your lower abdomen or groin, your back, your upper thighs, or your perineum. One mother says, "During labor, I sat cross-legged with an overstuffed hot water bottle at the small of my back. It felt great."

In many birthing-room and home deliveries, the woman's companion or birth attendant frequently applies hot compresses to her perineum to ease the intense stretching that takes place during the birth. One mother recalls, "Tim boiled hot water for the compresses which the midwife applied while I was pushing. This felt wonderful and I think it also helped stretch the vaginal opening. Even though I am an older mother (36) and had a scar from a previous episiotomy, I was able to deliver Bobby with only a superficial tear that did not require any repair."

Some Like It Cold.   For acute back pain, cold can be even more of a relief than heat. Use an ice pack directly on your back if that's where you're feeling your labor most intensely.

Try ice at the site of pain, anywhere between the site of pain and the brain, or on the side opposite the pain. Because of the gating mechanism in the central nervous system, intense cold at any of these locations may beat a pain message to your brain (see chapter 1). You might even apply an ice pack to the back of your neck for the duration of a contraction.

Cold's a good waker-upper, too, so ask for a cold compress on your forehead or a cool rubdown if you're feeling hot, sweaty, and tired late in labor. "The only way I could relax in labor," says one mother, "was to have a cold washcloth applied to my forehead."

Be prepared to try many different things in labor. You don't want to get so used to the same stimulus that it loses its effectiveness. Try cold alternated with heat because the variety may give you renewed relief.

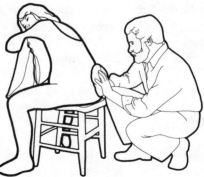

A hot or cold pack applied to the lower back can afford pain relief during labor.

But Not Too Hot or Too Cold.   When a woman experiences extreme pain (as in back labor, for example), she may be unaware of an extreme level of heat or cold. To avoid damage from burns or frost, anything that the labor partner cannot stand to touch should not be put next to the mother's skin. Placing a towel between the hot or cold pack and the mother's skin should ensure her safety.

Water Injections.   A new approach to water therapy, sterile water injections, has proven effective in two separate Scandinavian studies. Reporting in *Pain* and in the *American Journal of Obstetrics and Gynecology,* researchers described how intracutaneous injections of sterile water into women's backs relieved low back pain in labor.

Compared to control groups of women who received the placebo treatment, saline water injections, women who got the sterile water blocks reported significantly better pain relief after a brief initial burning sensation. This method may work to counteract the low back pain caused by the baby's posterior or forward-facing position by stimulating other nerve endings in the skin of the lower back.

Helpful Tools.   Your birthing place probably has a lot of the things you'll need for hot or cold applications. For heat, try a hot water bottle, warmed blankets, or hot compresses. Your partner can make hot compresses by soaking washcloths or towels in hot water and then wringing them out. You may want him to wrap the wet towels in a plastic bag and cover it with another dry towel.

He can make a cold compress by filling a sterile glove or plastic bag with ice chips and wrapping it in a towel, or simply by soaking a towel in ice water and wringing it out.

Many women swear by the plastic rolling pin that can be filled with ice chips and pressed firmly against their back as a relief for back labor. Ask if your hospital has one of these for your use during labor, or borrow one from a friend.

Hospitals frequently can supply reusable hot or cold packs for your use during labor. These are filled with a silica gel that can quickly absorb either heat or cold and will mold flexibly to your body, unlike a rigid ice pack. Such soft packs are available at most drugstores; if your hospital doesn't have them, you could buy and bring your own (see Resources).

10
Don't Take It
Lying Down:
Activity

How do you picture yourself during labor? Perhaps you've imagined yourself getting into bed, pulling up the covers, and simply lying there awaiting your baby's birth. Your husband mops your face with a wet washcloth while doctors and nurses flutter around your bedside. This image bears little resemblance to reality. If you really want to have your baby more quickly and with less pain, plan to get up and keep moving around as long as you can through labor. Since having a baby requires active participation on your part, you may want to prepare yourself to help the process by engaging in an exercise program during pregnancy. In your childbirth preparation class you'll probably learn several stretches to promote good posture and the proper functioning of the muscles that support your uterus.

You may also want to get involved in some regular aerobic exercise that pushes your heart and lungs to perform at their peak level. Aerobic exercise during pregnancy provides many benefits. It can build stamina, make you more comfortable, alleviate aches and pains, and relieve stress.

Aerobic exercise may even make your labor shorter and less painful. An American study published recently in the *American Journal of Obstetrics and Gynecology* reported that women who continued running or aerobic dancing during pregnancy enjoyed labors about 30 percent shorter than women who stopped exercising. Women who maintained a regular exercise program also required less labor stimulation and fewer epidurals, episiotomies, and cesarean deliveries. An Italian study in the same journal examined women having their second or third babies who pedaled on stationary bicycles three times a week for 30 minutes beginning around the fifth month of pregnancy. The bicyclists maintained higher endorphin levels during labor. Accordingly, they reported less pain than a matching group of sedentary women.

Even if regular exercise can't guarantee you a shorter or easier labor, it undoubtedly can help you to cope better with whatever labor has in store for you. Going into labor physically fit also means you will recover more quickly afterward.

The aerobic exercises of swimming, walking, and bicycling are readily available to most pregnant women. Or, you may choose to take an exercise class or purchase an exercise videotape (see Resources). Some women even continue jogging through their entire pregnancies. Be sure to get your doctor's approval before embarking on an exercise program, especially if you have medical problems such as high blood pressure. You should also be aware of the following precautions. The American College of Obstetricians and Gynecologists has established these guidelines to help prevent your core body temperature from rising too high and possibly harming your baby:

■ Keep your heart rate under 140 beats per minute during exercise.
■ Check your temperature by armpit or rectum at the end of your usual exercise to make sure it is less than 101°.
■ Limit very strenuous exercise to 15 minutes at a time.
■ Replenish fluids after exercising.
■ Avoid exercising outdoors in very hot weather or if you have a fever.

Walking through Labor.   Given freedom of choice, few women in any part of the world lie down during labor. The supine (flat on the back) position reportedly originated in the French court of Louis XIV. A voyeur who relished watching his mistress giving birth, the king's quirky preferences soon dictated fashion for the country. The supine position found almost universal favor in United States hospitals from the 1940s on because a woman's lying flat enabled her obstetrician to perform interventions such as forceps delivery, anesthesia, and episiotomy more easily.

But lying down has no medical benefits for most mothers. In fact, it carries several proven risks. When you lie on your back for long periods of time, the weight of the uterus compresses the descending aorta and inferior vena cava, blood vessels that supply or drain the lower part of your body. This interference with your circulation reduces your blood pressure, compromising blood flow to your baby and causing his heart rate to drop. When you stay upright (or at least off your back), placental circulation improves and fetal heart rate abnormalities may be alleviated.

A host of medical studies have demonstrated conclusively that upright positions shorten and ease labor. One famous Latin American study comparing reclining to vertical positions showed that labors for women who stayed upright were 36 percent shorter for first-time mothers and 25 percent shorter for mothers who had previously given birth. A British study comparing mothers who walked during labor to mothers who stayed in bed demonstrated that walking not only shortened labor but also reduced pain and the need for medication.

How does walking help your labor along? For one thing, your contractions become stronger, more regular, and more frequent when you stand up. Gravity helps your baby make his way through your pelvis. Furthermore, the upright position improves both the angle of your baby's body to your spine and the application of his head to your cervix. Because your uterus naturally tilts forward in your abdomen during contractions, it meets the least resistance when you are standing, leaning slightly forward. Finally, even though contractions get stronger when you're upright, many women feel more comfortable, more in charge, and better able to relax in this position. A typical mother put it this way: "When I lay down, it slowed my labor down in the early stage. When I was in active labor, I found lying down much more painful than when I was walking."

To promote your labor, keep walking as long as you can. One couple took a scenic stroll along the lakefront near their home before checking into the hospital when the woman's contractions were three minutes apart. Another mother remembers "walking and walking and walking around the apartment. During a contraction I would just hold onto something for support—a chair or my husband."

Because you'll probably need to rest while you're having contractions, learn to lean on your partner in a manner that won't make him sore the next day. Janet Balaskas, the author of *Active Birth,* suggests this as the best way for your partner to carry your weight properly: As you drape yourself around your partner, he should keep his shoulders down, bend his knees, and lean back slightly while tightening his buttocks. It's especially important for your partner not to bend forward with raised shoulders, because this will give him a backache.

Changing Positions during Labor.   Most women can't spend their entire labor walking around. Especially in a long labor, you may need to alternate walking with resting. Brief periods of sitting, kneeling, or side-lying can help you rest by temporarily reducing the strength of your contractions. Simply changing positions regularly will probably help you to be comfortable longer than any one "best" position you could find. One study found that obstetrical patients assumed an average of 7.5 different positions in labor.

Joyce Roberts, Ph.D., Professor of Maternal-Child Nursing at the University of Illinois at Chicago, has spent years researching positions for labor and delivery. Roberts points out, "A woman's contractions are most efficient if she alternately sits and stands during labor." It's also necessary, she says, to adopt positions that are comfortable and appropriate for your particular labor.

For example, you may need to be in bed because of bleeding, fetal distress, or premature rupture of membranes with your baby's head in a high position. If you have received an epidural, you have to stay in bed. If you are instructed to lie on your back, make sure your head is elevated with pillows and that you have a pillow or rolled-up blanket under one hip to tilt your uterus off your backbone. According to Roberts, alternating every half hour between lying on your back and lying on your side can help prevent the adverse effects reclining has on your blood pressure, your baby's heart rate, and your labor's progress.

Side-lying makes contractions less frequent than when you are standing, but they are also more efficient. Best of all, side-lying is good for your blood pressure. In fact, because it enhances circulation to your uterus, this position is often employed when a baby appears to be in distress.

As long as your labor is progressing normally, however, you may want to try any or all of the following positions in preference to lying flat, which tends to lengthen your labor and add to its risk and discomfort:

STAND, leaning against your partner, a high counter, or a bed.

KNEEL on all fours or with your arms and head against some pillows on an upraised bed. You could also try this on the floor, leaning on a cushion placed on the seat of a chair.

HALF-KNEEL, HALF-SQUAT, with one knee up and one knee down, in bed or on the floor. This is easier than squatting, described below. If it feels good to you, rock back and forth toward your raised knee during the contractions. Change legs as needed.

SIT UPRIGHT in bed or straddle a chair, leaning on a pillow on the back of the chair. A review of labor positions by the International Childbirth Education Association concluded that labor contractions were least efficient in sitting and supine positions. But sitting may still afford you a needed rest.

SQUAT on the floor or on the bed. When you squat, your pelvic outlet opens to its widest diameter and your contractions will be strong and effective.

Before you go into labor, you should practice squatting to build up your endurance. With your feet one and a half to two feet apart and your heels flat on the floor, descend gradually, without bouncing, and hold the squat for 15 to 20 seconds. Work up to holding this position for a minute at a time. If you have trouble keeping your feet flat, widen your stance a bit, or try putting a rolled blanket under your heels, or wearing low heels, or sitting on a short stack of books. Rise up slowly and repeat several times. If you need help balancing, lean against your partner or grasp a chair or bed. It's not a problem if your knees "crack," but don't do this exercise if you feel pain in your knees or pubic joint.

During labor you can vary the squatting position by squatting on the floor, leaning on a chair or on the labor bed. Or ask your partner to sit down on the bed or chair; facing away from him, try dangling into a squat, resting your elbows on his knees.

You could also squat in bed, supported under your arms on one side by your partner and on the other by a nurse. Or try squatting on the side of the bed with your arms draped around your partner's neck. Your partner could even sit behind you in bed, toboggan-style, supporting you under the arms as you squat. You could sit-squat on the low footstool in the labor room. Put a pillow and sterile pad on it, and just sit down with your knees higher than your hips. Or perch on a short pile of books, a large cushion, or a beanbag chair.

Look at the positions illustrated on the next page. Incorporate them into your practice of prepared childbirth techniques, so you can find out which ones are most comfortable for you and your partner.

One mother who moved around a lot during her labor remembers, "standing, holding on to the bureau, and literally dancing through the contractions. At times I would go from sitting to standing to all fours. My husband danced along next to me, wiping my face with a cloth, following me when I started walking, letting me hold on to him. During transition, I climbed on the bed and got onto all fours, then walked around again when the contraction was over."

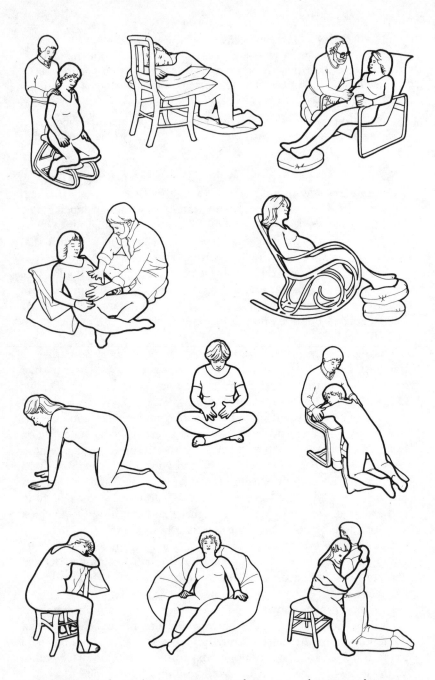

To alternate with standing, experiment with a variety of positions for comfort during labor.

You're probably wondering how you can do all this when standard hospital routines—fetal monitoring and IVs, for example—appear to command your complete immobility. It may not be easy.

You'll need to negotiate with your doctor well in advance of going into labor and come to a meeting of minds about the conduct of your birth. Many physicians insist on continuous electronic fetal monitoring and IVs in high-risk labors. But women may be monitored by remote control or on an intermittent basis, preserving their ability to move around. If an IV is medically necessary, it can be attached to a mobile pole, if your doctor agrees (see chapter 17).

If you learn that your hospital's or doctor's custom is to confine all women to bed for the duration of labor, you may want to express your own wishes and come to a compromise. It may be a good idea to have any agreement you reach entered into your chart, especially if your doctor might not be at the hospital while you are in labor.

You could plan simply to arrive at the hospital at a point late enough in labor that you are willing to get into bed. Or you may decide to switch to a birthing environment that respects your need to be comfortably active during labor.

Back Labor.   About three in ten women experience a labor in which continuous back pain accompanies the intermittent contraction pain. This situation frequently, though not always, occurs when a baby faces his mother's front instead of the more usual position, facing her back. In the typical position, the soft part of the baby's face "gives" and his mother usually does not feel significant back pressure until the latter part of labor, when the baby's head descends and presses against her rectum. But when a baby's skull is against his mother's back, there is no give; the back-facing or posterior position of the baby's head usually causes a severe backache for the mother until the baby turns. Labor may be prolonged as well as uncomfortable, because the contact of the baby's head to the cervix does not aid dilatation as efficiently.

To encourage your baby to rotate, try to keep moving. Don't lie flat on your back a moment longer than you must. With a baby's head pressing against your back, back-lying is especially painful. Vaginal exams requiring this position can be accomplished with your own or your partner's fists applying pressure into your low back.

Your baby's back will usually be a little more to one side of your spine than the other. You can ask your caregiver which side your baby's back is tending toward. If you choose a side-lying position, lie on the same side as your baby's back, with your upper leg raised on a pillow. Some women prefer kneeling, while others find the half-kneel, half-squat position mirrors the baby's asymmetry and offers comfort.

In the all-fours position, you might try pelvic rocking or swaying. Rock your hips to and fro, from side to side, or in small circles; these maneuvers will encourage the rotation of your baby and relieve your pain at the same time. Pelvic rocking on all fours may be especially helpful in turning your baby during transition or pushing.

Positions for Delivery.   When the time comes to push, a traditional American delivery team may still put a woman on her back. With her legs pulled apart and raised high in stirrups, she resembles a trussed turkey or an upended beetle. While a forceps delivery may require this position, known as the dorsal lithotomy position, it's an extremely ineffective one for a normal birth. Not surprisingly, this position results in a high incidence of spontaneous vaginal tears at birth. In fact, short of being suspended by your legs, lying on your back may be the worst possible position for having a baby.

Although it sounds "primitive," squatting is an excellent position for pushing. X-ray studies have shown that the cross-sectional surface area of your pelvis increases by as much as 30 percent when you squat. Aided by gravity, your expulsive efforts will be more effective. Your birth canal shortens and widens, too.

Even if you don't squat at the moment of giving birth, it usually takes a half hour to two or more hours of pushing for a first baby to come down to the vaginal opening. During the initial part of the pushing stage, you should be free to assume the position of your choice.

Because of its built-in associations with pushing, some women find sitting on a low toilet an effective way to squat during this stage of labor. Any of the squatting positions described above for labor can also be used for pushing. Indeed, a semi-squat, in which you dangle with your elbows resting on your partner's thighs, may be even better for you than the stationary squat, in which you support yourself on your feet. The dangling squat completely frees your pelvis to open in any direction, rather than locking it into a single position.

Squatting is tiring and uncomfortable when you're not used to it. What's more, you can seriously injure yourself by staying in this position for too long. So if you think you might try squatting for the pushing stage, remember to practice it beforehand and to sit back or lean forward into a kneeling position between contractions.

Many delivery beds now feature a "squat bar" that gives laboring women support while they push in a squatting position. A stainless steel rod, bent at a right angle, fits into the stirrup holes on a standard

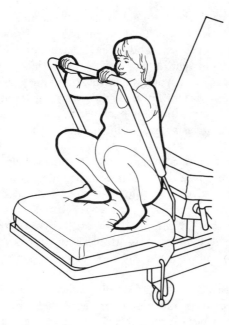

A delivery bed with a squat bar, which can help support you as you push.

delivery bed. A woman is encouraged to squat in a flat-footed position while holding on to the bar. At the end of each contraction, she lies back against a 45-degree-angle wedge to relax, or sits on a small stool, awaiting her next contraction.

You may not want or be able to squat while pushing. Don't worry about this. In fact, if your baby's head is not engaged when you begin pushing, squatting could prevent your baby from descending within your pelvis. Although squatting enlarges the outlet of the pelvis, it narrows the inlet or entrance to the pelvis. Squatting may thus prevent an unengaged baby from moving down into the pelvis.

Other positions can work just as well for you. Some women prefer to kneel or to get into the all-fours position. The all-fours position may aid the rotation of a baby who is coming down the birth canal facing forward. A hands-and-knees posture slows the descent of the baby, but this can be an advantage in a too-rapid delivery. It also allows your perineum to distend more gradually, which can reduce the need for an episiotomy.

A side-lying position also slows the baby's descent, but it's an efficient way to relieve back pain and certainly is better for you and your baby than lying on your back. One woman, in fact, found side-lying so comfortable for pushing that she asked her doctor to let her remain that way for delivery, and he did. She couldn't see the birth in this position, but was relieved not to have to sacrifice her comfort.

Sitting semi-upright on your weight-bearing bones, with your back rounded and knees drawn up, and with your legs bent and relaxed apart, is also a good position for pushing. Because it allows the sides of your pelvis to spread apart, it offers some of the same advantages as squatting.

Most labor beds now convert to delivery tables, helping you avoid that awkward move to a different bed in the midst of pushing. On the delivery table, your back should be well-supported by the table's upraised back, or by pillows or a wedge. Round your back into a C-shape, rather than arching it backward. Giving birth in a semi-upright position feels more comfortable and affords you better eye contact with your newborn when he is placed against you after the delivery.

If stirrups must be used, they should be lowered to a comfortable position. Many delivery tables now are equipped with footrests that allow your feet to rest comfortably lower than they can in conventional stirrups.

Staying active during labor—moving to keep yourself comfortable and to advance the birth process—is one of the best tools you have to reduce labor pain. But it may require a bit of advance preparation. First, be sure to pave the way by discussing your desire to walk during labor with your birth attendant. Second, practice your breathing and relaxation techniques in different positions. Finally, prepare your labor partner to give you physical and psychological support. With these preparations, you'll be well-equipped to relieve pain as you move your labor along naturally.

11
Everything But the Kitchen Sink:
Comfort Devices to Bring to the Hospital

"Something old, something new, something borrowed, something blue," are traditional items to bring to your wedding. When you have your baby, you'll want to bring special things with you, too—things that will make you more comfortable during labor.

Your childbirth educator will probably give you a list of items to bring to the hospital. To avoid carrying a tremendous satchel, ask your doctor or the nurse on your hospital tour which items the hospital has and which you should bring. For example, most hospitals have hot water bottles and ice packs. Some hospitals even have the kind of rolling pin you can put chopped ice into for a soothing back labor massage.

Pillows.   You'd think a hospital would have plenty of pillows, and, in fact, most hospitals do—if, that is, there aren't too many women in labor at the same time. If you go into labor at a popular time, pillows may have to be rationed, and you'll wish you'd brought some extras from home.

For supporting your body and allowing you comfort in many different positions, nothing beats having a luxurious supply of pillows.

One mother said, "I could have used five more pillows, the hospital bed was so uncomfortable."

Some women favor battery-operated vibrating pillows, some purchase inflatable pillows made especially for pregnant women, and some even buy pillows designed for body support during massage (see Resources). But regular bed pillows will do fine. In fact, the familiar smell of your own pillows may help you feel more relaxed in a foreign environment. Bring pillows covered with bright cases to distinguish yours from the hospital's. Pillows can even make your trip to the hospital more comfortable; put one on your lap to support your arms. One woman says, "I brought several pillows and blankets in the car and just reclined the seat as far back as it would go."

Focal Point.   Some women like to keep their eyes closed during labor, but many women appreciate having something beautiful to look at. A focal point can alleviate pain by taking away some of your ability to concentrate on it. In *Hello, Baby*, a popular movie about childbirth, one woman looks at a picture of her cat. Many women use flowers (as the flower opens up, so do they), a poster with a beautiful picture, or a picture of a baby. One mother chose the flower baby's breath, and says, "I found small, countable objects the most valuable focal point." Another woman had a poster with the message "Get Tough" on it. She says, "That really helped me when it started to hurt more."

You may not have any control over the way your labor room looks, but what you look at can have a bigger influence on you and your labor than you might think. A study done on postsurgical patients in a small Pennsylvania hospital showed that patients looking out their windows onto a tree view recovered faster and used fewer potent painkillers than did patients who looked out their windows onto a brick wall. The patients in the "wall" group and the patients in the "tree" group were identical in every way except for the views from their hospital windows. A beautiful or meaningful picture may have a relaxing effect on your body that will allow you to feel less pain, just like the patients who looked out at trees.

You needn't confine your focal point to a visual one. You might also choose an object with a pleasant aroma, such as a potpourri. One mother said, "Whenever I had a contraction, I just breathed in the scent of the potpourri." Just bear in mind that many women are quite sensitive to smell during labor.

Something to Apply Counterpressure, Heat, or Cold.   Because back pain in labor is so common, it's a good idea to have something with you to apply pressure to your lower back. Here are some commonly suggested items:

- A hot water bottle.
- A heating pad.
- An ice pack.
- A frozen picnic pack and a heated picnic pack, each wrapped in foil.
- A rolling pin or paint roller.
- A can of tennis balls or a couple of tennis balls in a nylon stocking.

Something to Ease Friction during Massage.   Bring along talc or cornstarch if you like to do effleurage (light massage) on your abdomen. For a kneading massage, bring unscented oil and a couple of soft towels. You may choose oil with a pleasant smell, but since women in late labor are often very sensitive to smells, it may be safest to avoid scent altogether.

Something for Your Dry Mouth.   Be sure to find out exactly what your doctor's procedures are regarding eating and drinking during labor. If it's OK, bring a thermos with an iced drink or hot sweetened raspberry leaf tea (see chapter 6). In most hospitals, you'll be permitted popsicles or sour lollipops (sweet ones tend to make you more nauseated). These can give you a little energy, and moisten a dry mouth. Your dry lips will also appreciate vaseline, lip gloss, or lip balm.

Hospitals always have washcloths, but you may want to bring your own to moisten your lips between contractions. Some women bring a couple of small sponges, such as makeup sponges, in a thermos of ice water for this purpose. You'll also appreciate having mouthwash or a toothbrush and toothpaste to relieve a sour mouth from long hours of labor or from a bout of vomiting.

Something to Keep You Cool.   Often during labor, your face gets flushed and sweaty. It's nice to be wiped off with a cool washcloth or to get a refreshing mist from a plant spray bottle; some women like a cool breeze from a portable fan or even from one made out of folded construction paper. One mother said, "I didn't want to be touched, but I enjoyed having my forehead and face continually wiped with a cool, wet towel."

If you have long hair, bring a hairbrush and something to hold your hair out of your face.

Something to Keep You Warm.   Cold feet can be uncomfortable during labor. A pair of warm socks should be in your bag of goodies to take to the hospital. The washcloths you've packed to keep your mouth moist and your forehead cool can also be soaked in very warm water and applied against your perineum while you're pushing.

Something for Your Labor Partner.   Nurses are usually wonderful about getting food trays and coffee for your labor companion, but come prepared in case you're laboring in the middle of the night or the staff is very busy. Even if the hospital cafeteria is open, you may not want your partner to leave you in the middle of labor. Therefore be sure to pack a high-energy snack for him—something you can stand the smell of while pregnant—a thermos of coffee if he drinks it, and breath mints or freshener.

A Mixed Bag.   Pack a paper bag to breathe into in case you hyperventilate from breathing too rapidly and deeply while tense. A surgical mask available in the hospital can be even easier to use, but bring the bag along just in case you can't get a mask when you need one.
　　You should also bring:

- Phone numbers of people to call after the baby is born.
- Change or credit cards for the phone calls.
- Your camera with film (if flashes aren't allowed in the delivery room, be sure your film is high-speed).
- Cards or games to pass the time if your labor is very long.
- Any review sheets or literature you've received from your childbirth teacher.
- A watch with a second hand for timing the contractions.
- A pencil and paper for taking notes.
- A cassette tape recorder or radio for music (see chapter 14).
- Glasses or contact lenses so you can see your baby's birth.
- Slippers to walk the halls.
- A mirror to watch as you push your baby out.
- A swimsuit for your partner to join you in the shower.

12
Listening to Your Body:
Biofeedback

Biofeedback is information about your body that you can use to improve your health or comfort. It can be as simple as having your labor partner check your muscle relaxation, listening to your own vocalizations, becoming aware of your position and breathing patterns, or watching your baby's head emerge. You will probably use many of these simple forms of biofeedback to get information about your condition during labor.

Instruments can provide biofeedback, too. In fact, you get instrumental biofeedback every time you step on a scale or read your temperature on a fever thermometer. During labor you may use the electronic fetal monitor to note your contractions and your baby's heartbeat.

When most people hear the word biofeedback, they think of an exacting training program that teaches you to monitor heretofore hidden processes like your blood pressure, muscle tension, and skin temperature. In fact, this kind of professional biofeedback training program may be useful for your pregnancy or labor.

For example, some women find themselves unable to achieve relaxation despite diligent training and practice. Dr. Joseph Barr, past president of the Illinois Biofeedback Society, suggests that biofeedback training can help the following women in pregnancy:

- A woman who cannot learn to relax using noninstrumental methods.
- A woman who had a particularly difficult first labor.
- A woman with a history of anxiety attacks.
- A woman who describes herself as high-strung or nervous.
- A woman who suffers from colitis, irritable bowel syndrome, or frequent tension headaches.

Some experts recommend biofeedback for pregnant women who prefer to control medical problems without medication. Bonnie Nusbaum-Jones, for example, had a history of migraine headaches so severe they required her take a medication that can induce miscarriage. When she was pregnant with her first child, she enrolled in biofeedback training at a headache clinic in a local hospital. "The training was extensive," she recalls. "They took me through every single part of my body to diagnose where I held tension and they explained the times that are most tense, like driving, and how to relax when I was inadvertently holding on to tension. I even got a complete psychological test.

"The machine I used primarily measured temperature change in my fingers. It took a lot of control and motivation to keep practicing what I learned, but it really helped my headaches. It also helped during childbirth. I took Lamaze classes, too, and I found that what I had learned from the biofeedback training enhanced my ability to concentrate, relax, and breathe during labor."

How Biofeedback Works

Biofeedback teaches people to become aware of very subtle changes in bodily functions. Before biofeedback was introduced in this country in the late 1960s, these functions were not believed to be under conscious control. As one researcher put it, without information about what your body is doing, you are like a blindfolded basketball player who has no opportunity to change his responses and improve his performance. With the information derived from biofeedback, however, you may learn to influence your body toward healthier responses. The information alone does not change your body's functioning, but teaches you to be more sensitive to your body's signals. Eventually you learn to substitute positive responses for less healthy ones.

Biofeedback training works particularly well for people who suffer from stress-related illnesses. It also helps patients who suffer from chronic pain—even children as young as three! Biofeedback provides chronically ill children a much-needed sense of mastery and competence over their bodies.

If you took biofeedback training, you would sit in front of a small electronic device with a panel of dials and lights. Electrodes attached from the machine to various parts of your body would determine subtle levels of neurological activity. This information would register instantaneously and be relayed to you by means of a visual or auditory signal—perhaps a light flashing or a tone beeping at a variable pitch—giving you immediate knowledge of the processes going on inside your body. With the guidance of a biofeedback therapist, you would then learn to influence your neurological activity by trying different relaxation strategies. You would be able to determine quickly which strategies work the best to modify your biofeedback signals and change your neurological activity in a positive direction.

The two most popular types of biofeedback equipment are the electromyograph and the thermograph. The electromyograph registers muscle tension by means of electrodes most typically placed on the forehead. On the assumption that a tense person will usually have colder extremities, the thermograph measures skin temperature at the extremities by means of a tiny sensor. Because this sensor registers changes in temperature of one one-hundredth of a degree, you can be trained to become aware of very slight changes.

To check your skin temperature on your own, you might want to purchase tiny, microencapsulated liquid crystals that change colors in response to fluctuating body temperature. "Bio Dots" can be purchased by mail from ICEA and "Stress Dots" are available from Choices through Communication Unlimited (see Resources). These inexpensive, disposable dots don't register the subtle changes visible on a thermograph, but they can help you train yourself to keep your hands warm and relaxed.

If high blood pressure troubles you during your pregnancy, you could use a device which allows you to become aware of your blood pressure and to lower it. Less frequently used biofeedback devices are the electroencephalograph, which monitors brain waves, and the galvanic skin response, which measures changes in sweat gland activity and is used for lie detection.

Which device should you use? After a screening interview with a biofeedback therapist, you would probably be advised to try a particular machine. The electromyograph is usually recommended for people who tend to respond to stress and pain by clenching their teeth. It's also for those who get tension headaches, back pain, or shoulder pain.

The thermograph, on the other hand, is especially effective for people who have vascular disorders such as migraine headaches or high blood pressure. Many people receive training on both machines.

After you are hooked up to your machine, you should receive detailed instructions on different relaxation strategies until you can work on your own. In general, the electromyograph works best with progressive relaxation techniques (see page 57) and the thermograph with autogenic training (see page 66).

Biofeedback training is not something you can do in the clinic and simply forget about when you return home. For this therapy to have any worthwhile effect, you need to practice what you've learned at least once or twice a day for a period of a half hour or more. Bonnie Nusbaum-Jones says, "I went to the clinic once a week for several months and I had to practice at home every day for at least a half an hour on a borrowed machine. It took a lot of control and motivation to keep up with the practicing. To learn to relax was easy, but putting it into effect in my daily life was more difficult. It's really work and it takes time."

Some studies suggest that biofeedback can reduce labor pain. One study, cited by Barbara A. Brown in *Stress and the Art of Biofeedback*, found a significant improvement in labor for women who trained in biofeedback and used it in labor compared to women who did not. Another study, reported in the *American Journal of Nursing*, contrasted 20 women who learned electromyographic biofeedback when they attended childbirth classes to 20 women who took classes without biofeedback. The biofeedback group practiced relaxation with the machinery 20 to 30 minutes a day for the six weeks of training, and kept up their skills by continuing to practice a few minutes a day until delivery. These women reported significantly lower levels of pain during labor, took fewer epidurals, and enjoyed shorter labors than the control group.

Yet, there may be limits to how much biofeedback can help. Ian St. James-Roberts and his colleagues at Queen Charlotte's Hospital for Women found that while electromyographic biofeedback techniques were useful in early labor, they did not postpone the onset of extreme pain or help the women cope better later on. Melzack and Wall suggest that biofeedback machinery is unnecessary and that women can learn relaxation as effectively without the machines. They point out that biofeedback itself does not relieve pain, but that the distraction, suggestion, relaxation, and sense of control stemming from the training do.

If you can achieve the effect you're looking for without the training, biofeedback is probably superfluous for you. But if you find it impossible to learn relaxation by other means, biofeedback may be an avenue you'd like to explore further.

Like any other therapy conducted by well-trained professionals, biofeedback does not come cheaply. The equipment is expensive, as is the therapist's time. Costs may range from $50 to $150 per session, depending on whether your therapist is a doctor, psychologist, or nurse, or a trained technician working in a clinic under the supervision of a health-care professional. Most people require between six and 12 sessions.

What you pay will also vary depending on how much help you need. If you can work with a relaxation tape and the machinery on your own you will pay less than if you need intensive work with the therapist. Your insurance policy may cover a substantial percentage of the cost, especially if your doctor prescribes biofeedback for a medical problem like migraines or high blood pressure. Some insurance policies will cover psychological services, so check to see whether behavior therapy is covered under your policy.

Selecting a Biofeedback Therapist

Ususally, biofeedback therapists are associated with large educational or health-care organizations. Your doctor may be able to give you a referral, or you may have to search on your own. In a large city, you can find biofeedback in the yellow pages. Psychology and psychiatry departments in universities may have biofeedback clinics. Frequently, psychologists, psychiatrists, osteopaths, chiropractors, and social workers in private practice use biofeedback as a mode of therapy. You can also write the Association for Applied Psychophysiology and Biofeedback (see Resources) to get the name of a local affiliate member.

Your biofeedback therapist may be a licensed professional in a field such as psychology or social work, or may be a trained technician working under such a professional. The advantage of going to a professional is that he or she may be more able to help you understand possible roadblocks to your progress. On the other hand, a technician sometimes has more time to spend with you, especially if he or she is not distracted by many other duties and responsibilities.

The person who helps you with biofeedback should not only be familiar with the instruments you are using; he or she should also be a good "advertisement" for the product. It's important that you feel comfortable with this person. "Vibes, rapport, and good chemistry are as important here as they are in any therapy," biofeedback expert

Dr. Joseph Barr advises. "Even if you can't put your finger on it, if it just doesn't feel right to you, that could easily get in the way of your learning the biofeedback skills."

Since people vary so widely in their physiological responses, look for a therapist who will adapt the training to your particular needs. Barr explains, "A good biofeedback therapist will put the person on the equipment for a few minutes and then ask, 'Are you more aware of images, sounds, or sensations?' People are each sensitive to different things, so as I guide them through relaxation, I usually customize people's instructions to give them what they find most effective."

The Electronic Fetal Monitor as a Biofeedback Device

During labor, you may be hooked up to an electronic fetal monitor, a device which registers your contractions and your baby's heartbeat simultaneously. Many women use this machine as a biofeedback tool to enable them to cope with the contractions. Here's how.

The external monitor senses the contractions by means of a device held in place by a thick elastic belt fastened at the very top of your abdomen, where your uterus begins its contraction. Though you don't ordinarily feel the contraction until it gets down to your cervix, the machine detects the contraction at the fundus, or top, of your uterus, and begins displaying it on a terminal or printed strip. The contraction may therefore be visible on the electronic fetal monitor before you can feel it yourself.

One mother said, "It really helped because I could 'see' the contractions. Instead of Bob having to say 'fifteen seconds, thirty seconds,' etc., I could see the crest and knew when the worst was over. That helped more than anything. The nurse was about to disconnect the monitor at one point, but I asked her to leave it on so we could watch it. I also used it to tell Bob when to get ready to press my back again."

Another mother recalls, "Although the belts were a bit uncomfortable, I found the monitor useful in that Marshall was able to prepare me before the contraction started; he reminded me to begin relaxing."

Some women don't like watching the monitor themselves. One woman said, "I hated the machine knowing what was coming before I did." Still, your husband can watch the monitor if you want him to: "Watching the monitor myself seemed to make the contractions more painful," another woman reported. "But my husband told me when the contractions were starting and when they had peaked. This gave me time to take a cleansing breath and begin to relax."

In an induced or augmented labor, the electronic fetal monitor may be an invaluable help. Mothers whose labors are stimulated by Pitocin often find the rapid onset of pain very hard to deal with. Pain is always harder to manage if comes on suddenly. As one mother said, "Since the Pitocin-induced contractions provided very little time to prepare for sharp peaks, Will would watch for the contraction. He cued my breathing and this made all the difference in the world in my being able to work with the pain instead of being caught completely off guard."

13
Mind Over Matter:
Visualization, Hypnosis, and Therapeutic Touch

Coaches and athletes have long known that the mental rehearsal of a physical skill such as shooting baskets can improve your performance nearly as much as actual practice. When you visualize yourself jogging, throwing a dart, skiing the slopes, or swinging your tennis racket, your body reacts as though you had actually done the activity!

Visualization may be effective in treating illness as well. In *Getting Well Again*, O. Carl Simonton and his colleagues detailed how imagery could be used to combat even terminal cancer. Norman Cousins's *Anatomy of an Illness* described how the author freed himself of a serious degenerative disease by using laughter. In *The Power Within*, Wendy Williams related the stories of ten people who used the powers of their minds to overturn poor medical prognoses.

Because your mind and body work as a unit, what goes on in your mind will exert a profound effect on your labor. Labor pain is enhanced—some even say it's created—by fear and tension.

Indeed, a study published in *Obstetrics and Gynecology* in 1989 reported that women who experienced distress-related thoughts during the very earliest part of labor suffered labors that were longer, more painful, and more complicated than those of women whose earliest labor thoughts centered on coping skills. Penny Simkin, who assists at births in the Seattle area, asks her childbirth students who call her in early labor to tell her what is going through their minds. "If I hear distress-related thoughts," Simkin says, "I say, 'I'll be right there.' I try to help women to reframe such thoughts in a more positive way. For example, if a mother says her contraction feels like a knife, I try to get her to imagine it instead as the back of a spoon." (See Pain Transformation, page 143).

Rather than focusing on how much your labor hurts, you may choose instead to ease labor pain by a variety of psychological techniques that can stimulate your imagination positively. Carl Jones, author of *Mind over Labor* and *Visualizations for an Easier Childbirth*, calls visualization "the most powerful method there is to reduce the fear and pain of childbirth."

This chapter will focus in depth on visualization and hypnosis, on using the powers of your own mind to improve labor and reduce pain. It will briefly describe therapeutic touch, a method which employs the imagination of your labor partner.

Seeing with Your Mind's Eye: Visualization

If you've daydreamed, relaxed before sleep, had sexual fantasies, or found yourself fully engrossed in a thrilling movie or novel, you already know from experience how images can relax or excite your body. But most people don't realize they can actually create images to promote health. For example, women at high risk for delivering preterm babies have been taught to develop visualizations to prevent premature cervical dilatation. Some women visualize a picture of their uterus wrapped in a sweater with a sleeve closed tightly around the cervix; others imagine a cocoon closed at both ends. One woman developed her own image of an impenetrable forest, with trees growing so thickly that nothing could escape.

Getting Started: Meditation.   Before you practice visualization for a normal delivery, you'll need to be able to relax your body completely (see chapter 4). Next, you should hone your skills of concentration by practicing meditation.

Meditate in a quiet, restful environment with your body fully relaxed. Don't meditate immediately after eating, but you shouldn't be hungry, either. Fifteen minutes at a time once or twice a day is about right for the beginner.

You can meditate on a physical object like a burning candle or a flower; a word, sound, syllable, or phrase; music; or your own breath. The purpose of meditation is to learn how to focus your thought on one thing.

The biggest roadblock will be those extraneous thoughts that crop up in your mind just when you're trying to concentrate on something else. You can deal with these thoughts in a couple of ways: Either resolve to ignore them, or simply be aware of them in a passive way. Some people like to think of the interrupting thoughts as clouds or birds that flit by and quickly disappear from view. If you can get past the inevitable miscellaneous thoughts, you'll be able to continue concentrating on your chosen focus for meditation.

Just learning to meditate, without any other visualization practice, will be helpful. One mother said, "I was able to relax completely between contractions throughout labor; this was probably due to my habit of meditating which I've been doing for the past year."

Getting Started: Imagery.   Once you have the ability to relax and concentrate, practice using imagery that will make you more comfortable during labor. When you begin work on visualization, keep the following things in mind:

- Employ as many of your senses as possible to make each image more vivid.
- Practice frequently to improve your visualization ability.
- Be passive about it; just let the visualization happen rather than working too hard at it.
- During labor, begin using imagery before pain becomes severe.

Try both free and programmed visualization. In free visualization, you simply allow images to come to you. In programmed visualization, you plan beforehand to imagine something specific.

Free Visualization.   In the "ideal setting" visualization, you use all your senses to imagine a beautiful place. If you love the beach, for example, relax your body completely and then picture the beach vividly. Imagine all the sights—the water lapping at the sand, the bright blue sky, the fleecy clouds, the palm trees or mountains behind you. Feel the warm sand or the gentle wind, or yourself floating in the refreshing water. Hear the waves, the songs of birds, or the lulling sounds of your own relaxed breathing. Smell the water, the suntan lotion, or the wind. Taste the salty breeze or your favorite beach snack.

Now the beach may not be an ideal setting for you. In fact, some people hate the beach and will picture only the hot sand and the flies!

Your ideal place may be a ski lodge on a crisp winter day, or a tropical garden, a special room in your house, the top of a mountain, the autumn woods, or a seat at the symphony.

Whatever setting you choose, the idea remains the same: Pick a place or situation, real or imagined, where you feel particularly relaxed and secure and try to make it come alive with all your senses. The rich imagining of such a place can be a restful haven for you whenever you need it—when you're trying to fall asleep at night, when you're feeling tense, or when you're in pain.

Once you've imagined yourself in the beautiful setting, see if anyone else joins you there. Some women use the "special place" imagery during pregnancy to ascertain who they'd like with them at their birth (see chapter 15). If any particular color, pattern, smell, or sound recurs in your ideal place, use this information to choose focal points for triggering your pleasant imagery. One mother, for example, favored a particular beach in Hawaii. During labor, she used a terry cloth towel, a poster, and suntan lotion to help imagine herself back on her special beach.

Programmed Visualization.   In programmed visualization, you give your imagination an assignment. Several types of programmed visualization may be helpful during labor. The first, *pain-relief visualization*, was developed primarily for chronic-pain patients, but it can be used to relieve any type of pain or as a pleasant substitute for pain. In the second type, *end-state visualization*, you picture any positive goal in order to focus yourself clearly upon it. A third type, *birth visualization*, enables you to "practice" relaxing and coping with the strong physical sensations of your labor. The fourth type, *creative dreaming*, is a special type of visualization that makes use of your nighttime imagination.

Each person will find one or another visualization most appropriate. Some people love to come up with imagery while others find producing it more of a challenge. Some people find it appealing to transform their pain into something more positive. Others prefer to escape from it, and still others wish to embrace it directly. Some people want to handle their pain themselves; others, if they could, would hand pain over to their helpers. Find some visualizations that appeal to you and give them a try. Put descriptions of the ones you like on tape and practice them several times a day. Try practicing with some simulated pain, as suggested in chapter 5. Remember that to get the most from visualization you must be fully relaxed and in a comfortable environment.

Pain-Relief Visualizations

Pain Transformation.   When you are practicing simulating contractions, or when you are feeling uncomfortable, locate your pain. How exactly does it feel? Can you transform it into a more manageable sensation? For example, if it feels like burning, can you make it feel like strong pressure instead? Or if it feels like a gripping vise, can you transform it into a tingling sensation? If you have an image of the pain, can you change it into something you can cope with?

Another way you can transform the pain is to put it into a different body part. Simply take the pain and try to experience it someplace else (see Glove Anesthesia, below).

What color is your pain? If it's hot red or orange, can you transform it into cool blue or green? What do you need to cool it down?

What shape is your pain? If it's a knot, can you see yourself untying it? If it's hard and square, what would make it soft and round out the sharp edges? If it's a large ball, can you watch it grow smaller and smaller until it becomes a tiny dot and finally disappears?

Put your pain into a colored balloon. Feel it expanding, then let the air out until it is completely deflated. Or, let the balloon just float away, with all the pain inside.

Go right to the center of your pain and feel the rest of the pain dissolving around this point. Or, imagine the pain diluting and diffusing all through your body, then exiting through your skin.

Breathe in energy and oxygen and breathe out tension and pain. See the pain actually leave your body.

Find the most comfortable and relaxed part of your body and allow that part to expand until your whole body feels comfortable.

Put your hand on the place where you feel pain. Take a deep breath. Breathe energy right into the place that hurts. Breathe out the pain.

Imagine a glorious, bright light over your head. As you breathe in, draw the light right into your body. Now bring it to the tense or painful part of your body and allow the light to ease your pain.

Glove Anesthesia.   This technique is adapted from David Bresler's *Free Yourself from Pain.* Imagine in front of you on a table a bucket filled with a clear, odorless fluid. The fluid is a very powerful anesthetic that can quickly penetrate your skin to render any tissue insensitive to pain. At the count of three, lower your hand into the imaginary bucket up to your wrist. Feel your fingertips beginning to tingle as the anesthetic starts to work. Soon, the skin on your whole hand feels tight and tingly. Then your muscles begin to feel completely

numb. Move your hand around to make sure the anesthetic penetrates completely.

Now, at the count of three, put your hand on the part of your
body that hurts. The numbness from your hand transfers into your
body and your hand receives your body's discomfort. Repeat the
process several times, transferring the anesthetic to your body and
the discomfort first into your hand and then into the bucket. When
you're ready to end this exercise, just shake your hand and the normal feelings will come right back.

Self-transformation.   When you feel pain, transport yourself to your
ideal setting. Imagine it with all your senses. Find a place within your
special setting to let go of all your fear and pain. Find another place
here from which you can derive the energy and power you'll need for
labor.

If it isn't too threatening, imagine you are out of your body. Explore
the space around you.

Give Your Pain Away.   The following techniques are adapted from
Directing the Movies of Your Mind by Adelaide Bry. Originally developed for joggers, these visualizations can help you feel the love and
support of your birthing environment.

Imagine a large hand along your back supporting you completely
as you labor. When you are fatigued or feeling pain, just see yourself
leaning into the hand.

Picture a wire extended between two trees. This is your finish line
or goal. A harness around you is connected to the span by another
wire and you are drawn toward your goal just as though you were
on a fishing line, being reeled in.

Pain Acceptance.   You may prefer to visualize exactly what the pain
of your labor is accomplishing. One mother says, "I just pictured the
inside of me, the uterus pulling up and thickening like tight panty
hose being put on, the baby's head gradually descending through the
cervix. I kept imagining how each contraction was stretching my
cervix and bringing the baby closer with each one. What kept me
going was the thought that the harder and stronger the pain, the closer I must be to delivery."

Other mothers picture the cervix as a flower opening, or the contractions as large waves which peak mightily, but inevitably recede.
They imagine themselves floating on these waves, tumultuous at
times, but always with the promise of descent after the peak.

Your images may be entirely internal, or you could bring pictures or objects to the hospital with you for a visual focus to prompt your internal imagery. In many societies laboring women look at symbols of opening and release; flowers, keys, and uncorked bottles are just a few of the images women all over the world focus on as their bodies open to give birth.

End-State Visualization

In this visualization you imagine yourself in the future with your baby already born. The image of a positive future is particularly helpful when you find it difficult to relax between contractions during labor. Your labor partner, too, might want to imagine the baby during labor to get him over the rough times.

Allow yourself to relax deeply. Close your eyes and picture your brand-new baby in your arms. Feel the baby's weight and warm softness. Hear the baby coo. The baby's skin is silky smooth and smells delightful. You look down into your baby's big clear eyes and the baby looks right back into yours.

Fathers may prefer to imagine themselves with a slightly older baby or child, perhaps on a walk in the park. The object here is to stimulate you to focus on the reality of your baby who really is coming soon despite how endless labor may seem.

A positive image of the future can get you through hard times in the present. As one mother recalls, "I kept telling myself the pain was temporary and I'd soon be holding the baby. My husband helped by reminding me to keep picturing the baby in my mind."

Birth Visualization

Notice what happens to your breathing and relaxation during the following visualization, adapted from *Birthing Normally* by Gayle Peterson. It will be particularly helpful if you can tailor the visualization to your own special needs. Then put it on a cassette tape, being sure to include pauses between the suggestions so that you have sufficient time to relax.

Find a comfortable spot where you can rest undisturbed for about 20 minutes. Allow your eyes to close as you release tension everywhere in your body. Take as long as you need to do this. . . . Breathe slowly and rhythmically, allowing more tension to leave with each exhaled breath. Feel how you calm your body and mind with your breath.

Imagine your baby floating inside your uterus, the thick-walled muscular sack that has been your baby's comfortable home for so many months. The cervix, the neck-like portion at the bottom of the uterus, has stayed closed and will stay closed until your baby and your body are ready for labor.

A thick plug of mucus lines the cervix, guarding both you and your baby from infection. Sometimes, the passage of this mucus plug is your first sign that labor is beginning. Or perhaps your amniotic sac will break with a slow leak or a rapid gush of fluid. Or, your labor might start with contractions, which gradually become stronger as the hours progress.

Imagine your labor beginning only when your body is ready for this to happen. Picture your uterus contracting, getting shorter and thicker on top and the cervix thinning and opening more with each contraction until in many hours it is opened fully around your baby's head.

See yourself at home coping well with these early contractions, going about your normal activities or perhaps even sleeping through them. If you're awake, imagine yourself walking around as long as possible, which will allow the contractions to be more efficient at doing their job. . . .

Now the contractions are beginning to get stronger. You get through each one by relaxing and letting yourself flow with it. You don't think about the past ones or the contractions still to come, but just go with the contraction you're experiencing right now. . . .

Imagine a contraction coming now. You can feel it coming closer and closer. Let your breathing relax you as you feel an intense pressure in your groin and lower back. The contraction builds . . . and builds . . . and *builds* . . . and you breathe calmly and let it do its work of opening up your cervix. Now it begins to feel as though it's going away. Let your breathing slow down naturally and allow any tension to drain right out of your body.

Picture yourself as very strong and capable of coping with all the new sensations you'll be feeling on this very special day, your baby's birthday. Imagine yourself going to the hospital when the right time comes. See yourself very comfortable in the labor room, with caring people attending to your needs.

Let yourself imagine another contraction now, this one even stronger than before. It builds . . . and builds . . . and builds . . . and *BUILDS*. You can't believe the incredible intensity of this feeling, but you are able to relax and let your body do its work.

Before you have a moment to gather your energy again, another contraction is coming. It builds . . . and it builds . . . and it *builds* . . . and it *BUILDS* . . . until you think you can't get through it. But you keep meeting it with your breathing and you keep picturing your cervix opening wider and wider and wider. . . . Now it's finally beginning to diminish and you slow your breathing down and you allow your body just to melt right into its support.

Another contraction is coming right now. It starts with such great power, you need to work very hard to let it happen and not to fight it. And you breathe and relax and perhaps you look right into your partner's eyes. It's getting stronger now . . . and building . . . and *building* . . . and you can feel your cervix opening wider and wider and your baby's head coming right down into your vagina. And now you feel a tremendous surge of power as it becomes time to push your baby down and out your vagina.

Visualize for a moment the passage your baby must make, down through your vagina, and then around your pubic bone. Your vagina is moist and soft. It stretches just enough to allow your baby through, opening right up as your baby is pushed down from the thickened, contracted uterus above. This caressing massage of being pushed through your vagina is healthy for your baby, just what your baby needs to stimulate his first breathing efforts. As you get ready to push your baby out, think "open" and "out"; just release those supple muscles around your vagina.

Imagine a pushing contraction coming and greet it with your breathing and release. It's powerful and you join in with its power, feeling great satisfaction in your efforts. Picture yourself pushing in the positions that are comfortable for you and efficient for your labor. Your baby will come down some with each push, then will go back just a little bit after the push is over.

Your pushing contractions come and go and you have the strength to work with each one to push your baby down further and further and further.

Imagine now your baby's head right down at your vaginal opening. You feel a stinging, burning sensation. Just breathe and release. Allow it to be—your skin will soon become quite naturally numbed with the pressure of your baby's head. At this point, it's important just to let the baby's head be born very slowly, so pant, don't push, as you feel your baby's head coming through. The release is tremendous! Now you feel a gush of the warm amniotic fluid following the baby's head. Perhaps another contraction is needed for the baby's shoulders. Now at last you feel your baby against your skin and hear that cry and see those clear, beautiful eyes looking up at you.

Your uterus now will contract again—just picture it—to give birth to the placenta. See in your mind's eye the uterus staying clamped down very firmly; this may help to prevent you from bleeding too much after your baby is born.

Imagine now just holding your baby, the baby you've dreamed of for so long, in your arms. . . . It really won't be much longer before you'll actually be holding that baby. For a few minutes, indulge in a fantasy about how your baby will look and feel and how proud and relieved you'll be after the birth. . . .

Now, begin to come back to where you are, realizing that when the perfect time comes for your baby to be born, your body will know exactly how to give birth, and you will be strong and fully capable of working effectively with your labor, just allowing the birth to happen in the best way possible.

Again, become aware of your gentle relaxed breathing as you begin very slowly to stretch and move your limbs. When you do get up, carry with you throughout the day a refreshing sense of well-being and joyous anticipation.

Creative Dreaming

Most pregnant women have anxious dreams about childbirth. If you're having them too, don't worry. In fact, you may have an easier labor than a pregnant woman whose slumbers are less disturbed, according to a study cited by Patricia Garfield in her *Creative Dreaming.* Patricia Maybruck suggests that women who are assertive in scary dreams have shorter labors than those who are victimized. In *Pregnancy and Dreams,* she writes, "If you find yourself victimized in any of your nightmares, they may be showing you that you are too passive or submissive in some areas. . . . As you become more assertive in your waking life, you probably will begin to defend yourself from nightmarish threats—or at least ask for assistance from a friendly dream character."

Whether or not your dreams are accompanied by anxiety, dreaming of labor probably means you are preparing yourself to cope with childbirth in a sort of psychological immunization. Once you've dealt with this situation in your dreams it will probably be easier to manage it in real life.

If you'd like to get some nighttime practice in coping with labor, you might try the following method for inducing a dream. Relaxing in a peaceful place, formulate your intention to dream about childbirth in a simple positive phrase such as, "Tonight I give birth in my dream." When you're drowsy and close to sleep, repeat that phrase to yourself several times. Visualize your dream as though it were happening. Be patient. It may take several weeks to induce a desired dream.

After you dream of childbirth, consider the message you've been given. You might converse with your dream images right when you wake up, asking them who they are and why they did what they did.

Hypnosis

Though hypnosis is one of the oldest techniques to use imagery for pain control, no one theory completely explains everything that happens during a hynotic trance. It's generally agreed that hypnosis is an altered state of awareness in which you concentrate so intensely that you are highly responsive to suggestions and able to tune out distracting stimuli.

Many people believe hypnosis is akin to sleep. Indeed, the very word hypnosis stems from a Greek root meaning "to put to sleep." Yet you are extremely alert under hypnosis, and your attention is quite focused. James Lowry, an obstetrician who hypnotizes many of his patients for labor, says, "In an average day, most of us spend about 35 to 40 percent of our time in a light trance, turning off all the noise around us."

Hypnosis boasts several medical uses. Many pain clinics teach hypnosis to their adult chronic-pain patients, and it has even been employed successfully with chronically ill children. In fact, hypnosis has been used in obstetrics since 1823 and in surgery since 1821. But it wasn't until 1958 that hypnosis won the official sanction of the American Medical Association as a legitimate therapy.

Being hypnotized for labor and delivery offers one great advantage. It can greatly reduce or even eliminate your need for painkillers, with their potentially depressing effects on you, your labor, and your baby.

More than 35 years ago, Dan Langell, an elementary-school administrator whose hobby was magic, hypnotized his wife Lorraine for the births of their second and third children. Langell recalls, "Lorraine was a good subject. The first time I tried it, she went under rather easily. Then we just practiced it once in a while. I gave her a posthypnotic suggestion so that she could control labor pain. The suggestion was that when she closed her eyes and counted to three the pain would be blocked out for a short time; then she could renew the suggestion as she needed to. I didn't want to block her pain completely because pain serves a protective function. She used this all the way until the end of labor, and the doctor gave her very little medication."

Many writers have pointed out the similarity of hypnosis to a number of prepared childbirth techniques: the training in relaxation, the concentration on anxiety reduction, the use of controlled breathing, and the use of strong psychological suggestion to cope with pain. Dr. Marlene Eisen, a psychologist and practicing hypnotherapist, says, "In childbirth education classes, as in hypnosis, women learn to focus in a different way, to shift their attention to reduce pain."

Hypnosis for childbirth has some disadvantages, however. It usually takes a substantial investment of time, energy, and professional guidance. Robert Bradley, author of *Husband-Coached Childbirth*, asserted that, compared to the simplicity of natural childbirth, hypnosis was "like wheeling up a cannon to shoot a sparrow when a BB gun would have sufficed." Hypnosis is not generally available to pregnant women, and it could be quite costly if your insurance doesn't cover outpatient mental health care.

Most obstetricians don't care to spend the unreimbursed time it takes to build this special relationship with their clients. Dr. James Lowry, on the other hand, offers each of his patients five free group hypnosis sessions. He also spends many extra hours privately counseling individual women who are particularly fearful about birth.

You might choose to be hypnotized for your baby's birth if you feel you need a stronger suggestion than that offered in prepared childbirth classes, or if you have had a previous unhappy medical experience. One mother, for example, had suffered many traumatic surgeries as a child. When she got pregnant with her first baby, she said, "the terrible experiences I'd had with doctors triggered the idea that I'd be out of control during labor and that painful things would be done to me." At the suggestion of her childbirth educator, she visited a hypnotherapist four times.

You might also choose hypnosis because of an unhappy experience with a previous birth. One mother, for example, who took Lamaze classes for the birth of her first child, anticipated that by using Lamaze techniques she would be able to control her labor pain. She says, "I was strong willed and the kind of person who always completed everything I tried. But trying so hard to be in control was *not* helpful for me. I ended up with a cesarean section after 23 hours of hard labor."

"With my second baby," she continues, "I had a vaginal delivery, but I still wasn't able to relax; I was just trying too hard. Finally, for my third birth I took a class on hypnosis because I needed to learn to give up control—to confront the pain and work with it. In contrast to my first two births, during this labor, I'd think, 'Here comes another labor pain. It's a good pain. It doesn't hurt. Let's study it and see what it's doing.' I would visualize the baby moving down through the pain."

Dr. Marlene Eisen recommends that couples who want to work with hypnosis for childbirth begin visiting a professional hypnotist weekly in about their fifth month. However, some women don't need such a lengthy period to learn hypnosis; eight to ten sessions, or even fewer, might be sufficient for you.

Unfortunately, not every woman is capable of being hypnotized into a profound trance. Melzack and Wall estimate that about 30 percent of people can be put into a deep trance, 30 percent can be put into a moderate trance, 30 percent can be put into a light trance, and about 10 percent seem not to be susceptible at all to being hypnotized. A study published in the *British Medical Journal* noted that women rated as "good" or "moderately good" subjects who received hypnotic training during pregnancy received significantly fewer epidurals than did women who were rated "poor subjects."

Dr. Eisen comments, "Most people can be hypnotized, but not everyone can be hypnotized deeply enough for it to work as an anesthetic. A woman should have an anesthesiologist available and shouldn't be ashamed if she needs some help with drugs."

The percentage of women who can be put into a deep trance is about the same proportion of people who are placebo reactors, but hypnosis cannot be explained merely by the placebo reaction. The pain relief in a profound trance is much deeper than any placebo could give. In addition, the hypnotized subject knows that she is responsible for her own pain relief, rather than imagining dependence upon a pill or injection.

Jill Angel is one of the very small percentage of women who can be hypnotized so deeply that they can undergo cesarean delivery without any additional anesthesia. She has done so twice. Before her children were born, Angel had taken a Silva Mind Control class in which she learned meditation and relaxation techniques; however, before her first cesarean under hypnosis, she'd had no formal hypnosis training at all.

When she gave birth to her first child in Wisconsin, Angel had been working as a teacher of young, handicapped children. She says, "I've always thought a lot of handicapped children's problems occurred on the delivery table. That's why I was so concerned about my babies getting medication. I really didn't want anything at all; my goal was to get that baby out without having any drugs in my body.

"During our childbirth preparation classes, a nurse-anesthetist, Robert Tithof, came to speak and he noticed that I got really relaxed. He happened to be on call when the obstetrician decided I was going to have a cesarean after 33 hours of labor, and he suggested I have the cesarean under hypnosis. I said, 'Why not?' I know that the mind is so powerful it can ignore the pain the body is feeling."

Reflecting on this labor several years later, Angel says, "I'd been in labor for such a long time. I just wanted it to be over with. I knew hypnosis would work, I knew I could relax myself. I imagined being in one of my favorite places, to take my mind off of what was happening, and I didn't feel anything during the surgery. I had my eyes closed, but I was fully awake and I heard everything that was going on. When the doctor said she was a girl, I took a look, then just closed my eyes again and relaxed while they sewed me up. As soon as that was done, the doctor said, 'Hop on the hospital cart,' and I did. He came to see me afterwards and I just needed a couple of aspirins."

In a local newspaper article written shortly after Katie Angel's birth, the nurse-anesthetist and obstetrician commented on the uniqueness of Jill Angel's experience. The obstetrician, Dr. Paul Capelli, said, "It was the first operation that I had performed without benefit of an anesthetic. I knew there was no pain because if she had felt anything the muscles of her abdominal wall would have contracted." Robert Tithof, the nurse-anesthetist, called Jill Angel "one in a thousand and a perfect candidate for hypnosis."

When Angel was pregnant with her second child three years later and planning a scheduled cesarean, she attended weekly sessions with Tithof for five months before the surgery. She says, "Anticipating my son's delivery was harder because I was more anxious. I had more of a visual idea about what would happen during the delivery. Concentrating on relaxing was more difficult the second time because it was a longer and more complicated surgery. I'm not sure I'd want to go through it again, but I'm pleased with the way things turned out. My motivation in having hypnosis for my deliveries was to do the best for my kids rather than for any personal achievement."

To cope with surgery under hypnosis, Jill Angel needed to be in a very deep trance state, attainable by a minority of women. But even a lighter hypnotic trance can be very helpful to a woman in labor. Esther Kaplan-Shain, a psychologist, reflected on the hypnosis training she'd received for her daughter's birth. "During my training sessions, hypnosis was such a relaxing, soothing kind of thing—a state of almost being in a bubble. I didn't feel that relaxed in labor, so, initially, I was sure I wasn't hypnotized. But, looking back on it now, I think I really was. The training certainly allowed me to use my own resources and to use the space of time in between the contractions to relax so totally that I was just about able to sleep. Whether or not I was in a trance, hypnosis provided me with the result I wanted: a great labor and delivery."

If you learn how to go into a trance for labor, you can continue to use these skills after your baby is born. "Once a woman has learned the skill of hypnosis," Dr. Marlene Eisen says, "she can use it in many different ways, for example, to imagine her breasts filling with milk or her nipples not hurting." Esther Kaplan-Shain says, "I've used many of the hypnotic metaphors for soothing and relaxation since my baby was born."

If you'd like to try hypnosis for your labor, delivery, and postpartum, ask your birth attendant for a referral, call your local medical society, or inquire with the psychiatry or psychology department of your hospital. Most state governments do not license or regulate hypnotists, but at least two major professional certifying organizations exist to guarantee the qualifications of affiliated practitioners (see Resources). The American Society of Clinical Hypnosis reports that 15,000 professionals currently practice the technique.

Contrary to popular opinion, gullibility doesn't correlate well with a person's ability to be hypnotized. People who tend to be most hypnotizable are good at focusing their attention and at concentrating. They love to immerse themselves in experiences, and they have rich inner lives because of their active imaginations.

A lot depends on personal chemistry, too. People who are not easily hypnotizable by one practitioner may sometimes be hypnotized by another, or they may be more successful at hypnotizing themselves.

Classes on hypnosis abound in adult education programs throughout the country. Many popular books, too, give instructions on self-hypnosis. In *Hypnotizing Yourself for Success*, Dr. Lynne O'Neill Hook writes, "You must remember that the trance state is your trance. The hypnotherapist or the person guiding you is like the individual below who has the data you need when you are flying a plane. That person can give you information, but it is you who performs the takeoffs, the flying, and the landings. Once you learn self-hypnosis, you can do the flying without anyone guiding you from the outside."

Instructions on self-hypnosis always begin with a technique to promote deep relaxation, include a specific suggestion, and conclude with a method for coming out of the hypnotic trance. Whether or not you actually go into a trance, any of the suggestions in the visualization section of this chapter could be put on tape or repeated to yourself in a self-hypnosis session.

In *Seeing with the Mind's Eye*, Mike Samuels and Nancy Samuels suggest the following technique for inducing a hypnotic trance:

> Find a tranquil place where you will be undisturbed. (Rest comfortably in a side-lying position, your arms and legs bent and supported on

pillows.) Let your eyes close. Take a slow, deep breath, expanding your chest and abdomen. Pause a moment. Then exhale slowly, feeling your chest and abdomen relax. Breathe in this way until you begin to feel quite relaxed. As you become more relaxed, your breathing will become slow and even. You now feel calm and comfortable.

Feel your feet and legs. Imagine them becoming very heavy. Say to yourself, "My feet are relaxing; they are becoming more and more relaxed. My feet are deeply relaxed." Rest for a moment. In the same way relax your ankles, lower legs, thighs, pelvis, abdomen, back, and chest. Rest again. Then relax your hands, forearms, upper arms, and shoulders. Rest. Relax the muscles of your neck and jaw, allowing your jaw to drop. Relax your tongue, cheeks, eyes, and forehead. Rest. Enjoy the feeling of total body relaxation.

You are now in a calm, relaxed state of being. To deepen this state imagine yourself in an elevator. Watch the doors close. Now look at the panel above the door which indicates the floor level. Imagine that number 10 is lit up. Feel the motion as the elevator begins to descend. As the elevator slowly passes each floor, you will become more and more relaxed, going to a deeper and deeper level of mind. Now see the number 9 light up. You are deeper and more relaxed. See number 8 light up. You are still deeper and more relaxed. Now 7. Deeper and more relaxed. 6. Still deeper. 5. Deeper still. 4. Deeper. 3 . . . 2 . . . 1.

Now, if you like, give yourself a specific suggestion for visualization or for pain relief during labor. To come out, Mike and Nancy Samuels suggest that you "simply enter the elevator and allow it to return to the tenth floor, watching the numbers light up as the elevator moves gently upward. At the tenth floor, open your eyes. You will be at your everyday state of mind and feel rested, strong, and healthy."

You could put this or a similar text on relaxation on a tape. Between the induction and the conclusion, insert a suggestion that has particular meaning for you.

Therapeutic Touch

Therapeutic touch is based on the folk healing system known as "laying on of hands," in which the healer places himself in a meditative state; holding his hands just above the patient, the healer transfers energy to the patient to relieve pain or other problems. In this technique, the *healer* is the one who visualizes the problem and its solution.

Therapeutic touch is the special province of nurses. Among nurses, its "guru" is Dolores Krieger, a professor at New York University.

Krieger's interest in the subject stemmed from her study of the psychic healer Oskar Estebany. Krieger has since taught the technique to thousands of health professionals.

Jean Battaglin, a veteran Lamaze teacher, studied therapeutic touch with Krieger. Battaglin says, "People do not stop at their skin. If you're sensitive to the energy that radiates from people, you can work with it. To prove to yourself that this is something we're not just making up, move your hands apart and almost together about three or four times. You will be able to perceive an energy source in between your hands. It's there; it's radiating from your body."

Unlike the laying on of hands, therapeutic touch doesn't require religious faith on the part of the healer or the patient; it doesn't even require that the healer touch the patient at all. Rather, it's based on the theory that energy is transferred from the healer's body to the patient's.

In therapeutic touch, the healer first learns to center himself or herself by concentrating intensely. Then she moves her hands along the "energy field" several inches from the patient's body, in order to diagnose problems in the flow of energy. If problems are found, she "brushes" the congested areas with her hands to permit the patient's energy to flow more freely—"like smoothing out a bed linen," says Jean Battaglin. Then, she treats the areas that need help. For example, if a spot feels hot, the healer imagines a cool color, or if a spot feels sluggish, she may imagine the color yellow to stimulate it. Finally, the healer intuits that the session is over; this usually takes about 20 to 25 minutes.

You could learn therapeutic touch from a book. The classic treatise on the subject is Krieger's *The Therapeutic Touch*. She has since written another book, *Living the Therapeutic Touch*.

But it's probably best to learn from a trained practitioner. Some childbirth educators, nurses, and nurse-midwives currently teach therapeutic touch to pregnant women's labor partners. They point out that its basic concepts are very similar to prepared childbirth techniques.

For example, the healer's centering at the beginning of the therapeutic touch session is very much like the focusing and relaxing taught in most childbirth classes. One of the biggest benefits for the pregnant woman whose partner practices therapeutic touch is that when her labor partner becomes more relaxed and centered, he is better able to help her do the same.

Since labor partners frequently learn massage techniques in childbirth class, some childbirth teachers include therapeutic touch as one more method of using the partner's hands to help the pregnant woman relax. Jean Battaglin advises, "Sometimes, when your partner doesn't really want you to touch her, just move your hand in the area where she's tense."

Skeptics assert that therapeutic touch, like other psychic healing processes, can be explained merely by the patient's faith that the cure will work. But even if the benefits of therapeutic touch are "all in the mind," and do not involve an actual transfer of positive energy, we must remember that the mind plays a critical role in labor. Therapeutic touch may be one more method to help you relax and let your labor happen.

14
Charms to Soothe:
Music

Music's ability to soothe the savage breast is much more than just a poetic metaphor. Musical sound influences your metabolic rate, pulse rate, and blood pressure. It can relax your muscles and encourage you to breathe more easily, and it can reduce your anxiety by decreasing your stress hormones. Chosen with care, a musical accompaniment may help you manage your labor more easily.

"We brought a tape recorder with cassettes that we had painstakingly selected for the occasion, so I had beautiful music in the background throughout labor," says one mother. "It was very soothing and helped me to establish a good breathing rhythm. Our little girl was born to a Mozart string quartet and placed on my chest for me to hold. This was the most wonderful moment of my life."

Music has been an integral part of healing rituals all over the world since the beginning of recorded history. In this century, scientists have found that dental and surgical patients listening to music require less anesthesia, and recover faster than patients who have nothing to listen to but the sounds of the medical procedures being performed on them. Even runners on a treadmill in a laboratory found the exercise less stressful when it was accompanied by music.

Some mothers claim that music is even more helpful than a visual focal point in capturing their attention during labor. Indeed, two studies published in the *Journal of Music Therapy* concluded that mothers experienced less labor pain when they listened to music.

Using music during labor offers you three benefits. First of all, music calms your physiological response to stress, allowing you to relax and let your labor happen more easily. Second, the rhythm of the music can cue your breathing, slowing you down and keeping you calm. Finally, focusing your attention on music takes your concentration away from sounds that may be anxiety provoking, such as the sounds of other women screaming, or the noises made by the machinery or the staff.

Selecting the Right Music.   Before your baby is born, practice relaxing with and without simulated contractions to see how different types of music affect you. The right music for your labor can be anything you enjoy, because if you like the music, your body will respond by relaxing. "When I was in early labor," recalls one mother, "Rob packed the music tapes we'd gotten for the event: Vivaldi and 'The Big Chill.'"

For early labor, try something slow, soft, and familiar. Some people like "New Age music," with no discernible rhythm or melody, while others prefer music with a 3/4 or 4/4 beat to help pace their breathing. When you're in active labor and transition, you may prefer something more vigorous, with a distinct rhythm or vocals. For pushing, Atlanta-based music therapists Jody Kershner and Virginia Schenk recommend that your music be "the most dynamic, matching the mother's physical and emotional response." For delivery, you'll probably want something harmonious and lovely for the baby to be born to.

Choosing your labor music need not be difficult. Music store personnel are usually happy to make suggestions if you describe what you're looking for. For example, if you enjoy imagining yourself in a special place when you relax (see chapter 13), you might look for environmental music that creates atmosphere and sparks memory. You can also make tape recordings off your radio, CD player, or record player.

If you choose to work with a registered music therapist (see Resources), your first meeting probably would take place several months before delivery. At that time, you and the therapist would discuss your musical preferences. A music therapist usually provides a practice tape with which you can work on relaxation, breathing, and imagery. With your individual tastes in mind, the therapist probably would compile at least 12 hours of different music for you to use during your labor.

To practice your relaxation and breathing before labor begins, try using music as a focus for meditation:

> Listen to the music. Feel its power lifting you upward. Let each measure flow through your whole body, relaxing every muscle and joint. Feel yourself floating along with the melody, relaxing more and more deeply.
> Listen to the silences between the sounds rather than to the sounds.
> Let the music massage or bathe your entire body.
> Imagine that you are the instrument(s) making the music.

When you go to the hospital, bring your cassette recorder. Pack earphones if you like, or simply play your tapes for everyone in the room to enjoy. Doctors and nurses often react as enthusiastically to music as do the expectant parents. Music can soothe everybody involved in your labor.

Adjust the volume to your need, perhaps louder when a contraction begins and quieter between contractions. Rhythmic body motions in time with the music can add to your attention focus and provide even more pain relief. Tap the rhythm with your finger or foot, nod your head, or massage your body in time to the music.

One mother says, "I swayed back and forth rhythmically to keep relaxed." Another notes, "Along with the Lamaze breathing, I found it comforting to roll my head, weaving and bobbing from side to side. This gave me more relief than just thrashing about."

Whether or not you use music during your labor, you can concentrate on your own sounds to help you relax in labor. As long as the sounds you're making help you relax, they're probably a good idea. One woman says, "To overcome concentrating on the pain, I found myself singing part of each breath. This was very helpful." During a contraction, you might make a sound or hum in your throat on the exhaled breath. Imagine that sound melting your cervix open.

Sounds that *won't* be helpful to you are high-pitched screams or repeated cries for help. Hearing yourself making these sounds will probably just make you more tense. But moaning, or singing out with your breaths, can provide you with a release that will make you feel better. "Speaking the breathing, actually vocalizing the ah-hee, ah-hoo, seemed to ease my feeling of desperation," one woman said.

Using music in labor—giving birth by the "rhythm method"— gives you a positive focus for your attention, reducing your labor pain and making birth more enjoyable. "It was," says one mother, "a celebration of joy when our son was born. The music made it even more festive and special."

15
You Need a Friend:
Companionship

Giving birth is one of the most intense physical and emotional experiences you'll ever have. Likening herself in labor to a small boat in a storm, one woman writes, "My husband was my navigator; he just took command and steered me through. His reassuring 'You're doing great, keep it up, we're almost there,' and his breathing along with me—counting out my pace—enabled me to sail through intense contractions that would otherwise have tossed me to and fro in confusion and panic."

Since the early 1970s, when just over one-quarter of American fathers were present in the delivery room, the percentage has tripled. Today more than four out of five fathers assist their wives at birth.

Americans have only recently rediscovered the importance of a supportive labor companion, but it's hardly a new idea. In almost every traditional culture studied by anthropologists women labor accompanied by a companion.

In this country, too, birth used to be a communal event. But when the majority of American women began to give birth in the hospital during the 1940s, this traditional wisdom temporarily disappeared. Family members, and anyone else who was not a medical professional, were barred from accompanying the woman in labor. Except for the labor and delivery nurse who came in now and then to check blood pressure or administer medication, the laboring woman languished alone.

Childbirth education began in the 1960s to reverse this historical aberration. Now women who wanted to be awake for their babies' births could not only get the psychological support they needed, but could also share with their husbands the exciting experience of giving birth.

Typically, American women relish having their husbands with them during labor. Being together at birth fosters a very special bond between a couple. "Bob and I became like one person with each contraction," says one mother. Another recalls proudly, "My husband stayed with me through all those hours. He reminded me to breathe and to relax. He massaged my shoulders and my back. He held my hand and kept assuring me that everything would be all right. He also gave me ice and wiped the sweat from my face."

Husbands, too, often feel that they have been indispensable to their laboring wives. One reports, "I loved the work of a coach. Even during the slow times, it felt very right for me to be there with Tina. We felt such a strong sense of being in this together." Another father says, "I feel I played an important role in providing support and meaning to the entire labor experience."

Your Labor Support:
Husbands and Others

You probably know very well why you want to have your husband with you when you have your baby. "It'll make me feel less frightened to have my husband there," say scores of women on their first night of childbirth classes. "He knows me, he knows how to calm me down and how to comfort me."

Sometimes a woman can't anticipate just how helpful her husband will be. One mother writes:

> I remember thinking the coach's role wasn't really that important. I was glad my husband would be there; I knew that the comfort he could give me would be important, but I didn't think he could be more than a comforter. Was I wrong!
>
> I could not have had Charlie if Steve wasn't with me. He walked down the halls with me, suggested changes in position, or actions that would make me more comfortable, made me drink so I wouldn't need an IV, but, most of all, he kept me together during the active and tran-

sitional phase. For hour after hour Steve took every breath I took. He shook me to wake me up, told me to open my eyes. Honest, I was helpless. And then to have him by me while I was pushing was so important, too. He was indispensable.

"Mike did everything for me," recalls another woman. "He held ice on my lower back where the pain was. He breathed with me to keep a steady rhythm. He would warn me at the beginning of a contraction even before I could feel it. He knew that I didn't want to be talked to during the beginning or peak of a contraction because I was trying hard to concentrate on a focal point and my breathing. But as he saw the curve descend, he'd say, 'You're coming down now,' just as I felt the pain ease. It felt so good!"

In the 1960s and 1970s, when the medical establishment fought to keep husbands and other helpers out of labor and delivery rooms, researchers struggled to demonstrate tangible benefits of having a labor support person. Indeed, study after study proved that husbands did make a difference. Women whose husbands assisted them at birth experienced less pain, used less medication, and had more peak experiences at birth than did women who labored and delivered alone. One study comparing father and nurse support during labor discovered that fathers were much more likely than labor nurses to touch women in labor.

Not surprisingly, women's reports after birth usually claim that their husband's presence and practical help got them through labor. A typical woman writes: "Kurt was fantastic. He kept me as relaxed as possible, reacted to each stage with positive ideas, and kept me concentrated on a small time span. I couldn't have done it without him."

Some couples feel they would like to keep their child's birth as private as possible, and, for many women, having their husband as their only labor companion works fine. But some women have no husbands, others have husbands who are unwilling or unable to be labor helpers, and still others appreciate the extra support of a labor companion in addition to their husband.

In other parts of the world birth companions traditionally have been other women. In fact, in 81 percent of nonindustrial societies, men are not even allowed at birth. Anthropologist Brigitte Jordan describes birth in the Yucatan, where the husband *is* expected to be there, as an event that also calls forth a pool of "interchangeable qualified helpers." These helpers are all women who themselves have given birth and who can be relied upon to spell each other during a prolonged labor.

Today, many writers advocate the return of female birth support, suggesting that you bring not only your husband, but another woman or women as well. In their book of the same title, Paulina Perez and Cheryl Snedeker call labor assistants *Special Women.* The authors write, "When contractions are intense and the journey seems endless, it is often important for the mother to know that she is being taken care of by another woman who has been through the birth experience." Recent research bears out their advice.

A study of more than 600 women in labor at Jefferson Davis Hospital in Houston revealed that women laboring with the support of another woman had shorter labors and less than half as many cesarean deliveries as women who labored without partners. Compared to the control group, even fewer of the supported women used forceps, Pitocin, or epidurals for their births. In addition, their babies were less likely to need prolonged hospitalization.

Dr. John Kennell, professor of pediatrics at Case Western Reserve University School of Medicine in Cleveland, conducted this study with several colleagues. Trying to explain how such a simple intervention could bring such positive results, the researchers speculated that a supportive companion may reduce catecholamine levels by lessening maternal anxiety, thereby promoting uterine contractile activity and uterine blood flow. "Labor support is centuries old," the authors concluded, but "its positive benefits should not be overlooked in the trend toward more and increasingly complex technology."

Is female support necessary even if you're also bringing your own husband? It's hard to answer that question with certainty, but another recent study published in the *Journal of Psychosomatic Obstetrics and Gynaecology* suggested that compared to male partners, female labor supporters provided much more constant physical contact.

More than a decade ago, Dr. Kennell and his co-workers had studied women giving birth in Guatemala with and without a supportive woman companion. There, too, women with companions had shorter labors and suffered far fewer complications like fetal distress and cesarean deliveries.

At that time, Kennell commented about the importance of having a labor companion:

> Let me note that if I had told you today about a new medication or a new electronic device that would reduce problems of fetal asphyxia and the progress of labor by two-thirds, cut labor length by one-half, and enhance mother-infant interaction after delivery, I expect that there would be a stampede to obtain this new medication or device in every obstetric unit in the United States, *no matter what the cost.* Just because the supportive companion makes good common sense does not decrease its importance.

Pat Summers chose to have a friend accompany her and her husband when she was in labor. She says, "My husband is not the type to read books and study childbirth like I did. He would go to Lamaze class and practically fall asleep. I wanted him there to experience the miracle of birth, but I knew he just couldn't be the main person to help me through the labor."

Pat asked her friend Donna to come to the hospital with her and her husband because Donna had recently given birth to two babies without using drugs. "I needed someone there with me who'd be a complete advocate for the way I wanted my childbirth to go," says Pat. "I wanted no interventions unless there was a serious complication."

"My husband was relieved," she adds. "And, as it turned out, it was very helpful to have an additional person, because I had back labor from 3:30 until I delivered at midnight. The only way to counteract that was having someone rub my back continuously. No one person could have done that for eight and a half hours. Donna knew exactly how to rub my back to make it feel good, and my husband learned how to do it right by watching her.

"If it weren't for Donna, I know I would have taken drugs. When I asked for a shot of a narcotic, Donna was the one that said to me, 'You know you don't really want that. You're doing fine; hang in there.' Now when I'd first come to the hospital, I'd told them I didn't want drugs, but by then, a new nurse had taken over. That's why I wanted a friend there. Donna was a consistent person who could help me get what I really wanted. What's more, I'd wanted to stay home as long as possible, and I knew that she would come to my house and be with me whereas, of course, a nurse couldn't do that."

Hospitals aren't always hospitable to the idea of women bringing extra companions with them. According to a survey conducted by the American Hospital Association in 1989, 99 percent of responding hospitals allowed fathers in the delivery room, but just 68 percent permitted other friends and relatives.

The arguments against extra birth companions sound remarkably similar to arguments in the early 1970s against husbands accompanying their wives in labor. Before Pat Summers's delivery, for example, her doctor said he would prefer her not to bring an extra person, but "it would be OK if that's what I wanted. He explained, 'We get nervous about it because extra people hinder things and get in the way and cause problems.'"

Pat had to call the hospital twice to confirm the arrangements. She says, "At first, when I called the hospital, the nurse said my female companion had to be a Lamaze teacher. The second time I called, they just said I could bring anyone I wanted as long as she wasn't obnoxious. I took that as an OK.

"Donna wasn't intrusive with the hospital staff. She was just there to help me. She breathed with me and counted with me and pushed with me. And, after the delivery, my obstetrician said three different times, 'We ought to hire your friend; she was really terrific. She made the nurse's job easier by being there.' My nurse didn't feel left out either," observes Pat. "She played an important role in the birth. She answered questions, she talked about the fetal monitor. Each person there with me had a significant and different role."

Experts who advocate extra labor support cite experiences like Pat's to show that bringing an additional person does not mean supplanting the husband or the labor nurse. Instead, an extra helper can offer needed support to both the mother and the father and can make up for the inability of all-too-busy nursing staffs to give the one-to-one care women in labor need. After all, points out labor support advocate Beth Shearer, "The labor and delivery nurse comes and goes and has other responsibilities; rarely can she stay through your whole labor. Too, she's a stranger. It just is not human nature to put yourself in the hands of a complete stranger in times of stress. Your husband has an appropriate role at birth, but he shouldn't be expected to carry the whole role of supporting you himself. Everyone who has been in labor or sat with women in labor knows that it is virtually impossible to have too much support."

A woman who "mothers the mother" by helping out during the birth or afterwards may be called by a Greek name, *doula,* after anthropologist Dana Raphael's usage in *The Tender Gift: Breastfeeding.* Raphael writes, "We use the term 'doula' as a title for those individuals who surround, interact with, and aid the mother at any time within the perinatal period, which includes pregnancy, birth, and lactation."

A doula can do whatever you need during labor. Her functions usually include the following:

- She helps you find your own best methods of coping with labor.
- She relieves and supports the father.
- She nurtures you.
- She determines your best interests and advocates these to the hospital staff.

While a doula may be any person who supports you in labor, another type of labor companion, the *monitrice,* usually has professional training as a nurse. She may also be a childbirth educator or a midwife. In addition to supporting you during labor, a monitrice can also do some of the jobs of a labor and delivery nurse.

In *A Good Birth, A Safe Birth*, authors Diana Korte and Roberta Scaer suggest that you bring both a doula and a monitrice to the hospital with you. Because she's a nurse, your monitrice can examine you at home, enabling you to remain there longer. She might also listen to fetal heart tones by auscultation, allowing you to postpone or avoid electronic fetal monitoring. Most important, a monitrice can offer you the one-to-one nursing support every woman needs during labor, but that most women rarely get in today's busy and understaffed obstetrical units.

Beth Shearer worked as a labor support person in the Boston area for five years. "I supported about 175 births," Shearer recalls. "I always included two prenatal visits and a postpartum contact because it's necessary for women to process the experience. I did what people wanted me to. The job involves physical support—things like back rubs, encouraging women to get up and walk around—lots of emotional support, and advocacy in the hospital setting.

"Ideally," continues Shearer, "the labor support person would be someone you know, someone who's a part of your life. This breaks down in our culture because you don't always have people in your life who can fill that role for you. For example, your mother may not know how to support you in labor because she doesn't remember her own labor."

While Shearer advocates labor support for all women, she discourages women from using hired labor help to "protect" themselves from the hospital. "The most difficult thing for me to learn," she says, "was how to assert myself for the women without antagonizing the staff or the doctor. I'd tell my clients, 'I'll support you, but I'm not going to fight a pitched battle over your body.'"

As hospitals become more familiar with the use of labor supporters, staff resistance will diminish. For now, if you'd like to bring an extra labor companion, be sure you pave the way well before your delivery. In an article on labor support, Beth Shearer suggests talking to your doctor, then writing to the hospital stating your intent to have an extra support person, and, finally, bringing a copy of the letter when you come for the delivery.

Depending on your particular needs, you may choose to labor with your husband only; to bring a friend as Pat Summers did; to invite your mother, mother-in-law, or sister; or to hire a professional monitrice—your childbirth educator, a nurse, or a midwife.

June Shields loved having her mother with her during labor: "Mom hadn't been through Lamaze, but she knew with her motherly instincts exactly how to help. Both Scott and Mom helped me to relax and concentrate. It was fantastic having her there." Gina Ganz's sister had taken Lamaze and recently had her own second baby. "She assisted my husband in coaching and supporting me. When I pushed, my husband stood on one side and my sister on the other, each supporting a leg and reminding me what to do with each push."

Marge O'Connor made arrangements through her obstetrician to have a student nurse accompany her for labor. She was fortunate enough to inherit the student's instructor, too. "When the instructor, Lucy, walked into the room," recalls Marge, "you could see that she knew exactly what she was doing. I had back labor, and when Joey's head descended, it felt as though someone inside was pushing his cleats against my spine; it was intolerable. Lucy came in and she was so calm. She just gave off this aura of 'I know about this; there's something we can do.' She used both hands, the heel of one hand and the other hand on top, to push hard and move the bone away from Joey's head. She taught the nursing student and my husband how to do this. And when someone was doing it right, it was just labor instead of agony."

After having her own baby, Marge eagerly volunteered to coach a friend whose husband was unable to take an active role in her labor. Marge says, "At one point when Ann was in transition she was in a lot of pain. And she asked me, 'Does it get any worse than this?' Of course, I couldn't really be sure, but I took a chance and said, 'No, it's different when you're pushing, but it never gets any worse than this—you've reached the maximum.'" This reassurance rings true when it comes from someone who's "been there," and it's a profound help to the laboring woman.

Some labor supporters combine the functions of a doula and a monitrice. You'll have to decide beforehand just what you would like your own companion or companions to do. Of course, your mother or your best friend will provide their labor support for free. But if you choose a professional labor support person, agree before the birth on either an hourly rate or a set fee for the entire labor. In the case of a private-duty nurse, your insurance company may reimburse you for part or all of her charge.

Finding Labor Support

Labor support services are available in a growing number of communities (see Resources). The women who work for these groups may be trained volunteers or professional monitrices. Your birth attendant or childbirth educator can usually tell you what type of labor support services exist in your community. Or call the International Childbirth Education Association (see Resources) to get the name of your state coordinator, who can refer you to local resources.

If you're looking for a monitrice, the authors of *A Good Birth, A Safe Birth* suggest calling the hospital's obstetric unit to see if they have on-call nurses. If private obstetric nurses are unavailable, call the director of nursing or the hospital administration. Since private-duty nurses often work on the medical-surgical unit, they should be available for labor and delivery. Childbirth educators will sometimes accompany their students to labor, and some are qualified to perform nursing tasks like listening to the fetal heart tones.

Whether you're thinking about hiring labor support or you're considering using a volunteer, the main question you must ask yourself is, "Does this person feel right to have around at birth?" As Pat Summers says, "I'd gotten a list of nurse-midwives and had called some of them, but I hadn't talked to anyone I really thought I could be comfortable with. Donna, my friend, was so enthusiastic about coming with me. And once I picked her I knew I'd done the right thing. I really felt good about it."

If you are looking for labor help, here are some things you should consider:

- What is this person's training and experience with birth?
- What are her attitudes about birth? Are they consistent with yours? If not, is she still prepared to advocate your goals for the birth to the hospital staff?
- What services are included? For example, will she attend you at home? Does she do internal exams? Will she listen to the fetal heart tones, give breastfeeding help, or do newborn monitoring?
- Will this person be available when you go into labor, and what are her backup resources if she isn't?
- Is she affiliated with and accepted by your hospital?
- Does she have references from satisfied clients?

It might seem as though the more birth companions you have, the more easily your labor will go. Then again, maybe not. Randi Ettner, a psychologist, has explored how women's chosen companions affected their labors. Ettner discovered, "The more people there are in the delivery room, the less likely the people are to be emotionally available to the woman. It also starts to set up some performance anxiety. Sometimes, it seems, women want people there because they don't trust themselves to be able to give birth. They think: 'I'll have so-and-so because she's a nurse-midwife,' or 'I will have so-and-so because she's a Bradley instructor.' They're relying on others rather than on themselves to get them through this ordeal. The women I saw who had normal deliveries had one or two supportive people with them while they labored and delivered, aside from medical personnel. Usually that was a husband and a friend, or a husband and a sister."

How to Help a Woman in Labor

If you're planning to help your wife or a friend through labor, have a good discussion beforehand so that you understand exactly what kind of help she expects of you during labor. "Get her feedback," advises Kathy Cain, author of *Partners in Birth*. "That way you'll know what she likes and doesn't like and you can perfect your technique together."

Try and attend childbirth classes with her and practice the prepared childbirth exercises together. You should also accompany her on a tour of the hospital or birth center to familiarize yourself with the staff and environment you'll encounter during labor.

After this basic preparation, working with a woman in labor is really more an art than a science. Your most important qualities will be a desire to share the birth experience and a willingness to do what helps the woman most at the time.

Make an effort to stay relaxed and comfortable. "Carry a packed bag of food with you to the labor room," warns one father who didn't. "If it's nighttime or your wife wants you not to leave, you can become terribly hungry." When you do have to leave your partner to go to the bathroom or to get a snack, be sure to get a substitute to help her out while you're gone. Wear your most comfortable shoes and clothes, and use good body mechanics so you don't get a backache when you're massaging or supporting your partner.

Stay positive in all your communications to the laboring woman. Of course, you shouldn't deny her pain. But it doesn't help her for you to be overwhelmed by it, and she doesn't need you to save her from it either. What she does need from you is this acknowledgment: what she's feeling is hard, but it's also normal, productive, and positive. In fact you can reassure your partner that the more pain she feels, the closer she probably is to having her baby.

A woman in labor may need your active help if she is to do the relaxation and breathing which will make her feel better. "Joan sat on the edge of the bed and lost it," recalls one father. "When she began to cry, I felt really needed. I picked her up and dusted her off;

then I helped her with the concentration, relaxation, and breathing. We breathed together and mastered it."

Each woman's needs will be somewhat different. Some women want strong, active participation from their partners throughout. One husband says, "For the last five hours of Gail's labor, I was indispensable. I massaged her back, breathed with her, read the monitor, coaxed her, supported her for every minute. The only thing I didn't do was feel her pain."

Other women may want to cope with labor on their own. One mother says, "I didn't like my husband to do anything to break my concentration. I needed to feel his presence, but not see or hear it." Her husband says, "Until I realized that she wanted to use her own inner strength to cope, I was probably not helping by trying to help too much."

Your partner's needs may change in the course of labor, and, as the support person, you'll have to be sensitive to her changes. A woman who wanted to handle labor alone in the beginning says this:

> Through most of active labor, I withdrew inward. I didn't want to answer any questions or open my eyes. I simply lay on my side and relaxed as if going to sleep and breathed slow breaths through each contraction. My husband got the message that I didn't have any desire for his help during this phase and lay down on the couch for a nap. This worked out well to fortify him for later when I really needed him.

You may want to try some of the imagery from chapter 13 to let the woman know what is going on with her body and to help her relax completely between contractions. But a woman in labor doesn't always need or want words from her labor partner. Your gestures, the way you massage her, take her hand, mop her brow, or firmly hold her when she needs to be held can all communicate your presence and love without any words at all.

In *The Birth Partner*, author Penny Simkin comments, "Many couples develop their own 'rituals' for handling the mother's contractions; that is, they repeat the same series of comforting actions with each contraction." These rituals cannot be planned in advance, but if you discover a particular way of touching or holding your partner that's soothing, keep repeating it as long as it works, and then try something different.

Toward the end of labor many women become quite discouraged and need active help from their labor partners. If your partner panics, you may need to call her by name to get her attention. Stand very close to her as you lock eyes and work together. One mother recalls, "My husband was my focal point and he breathed along with me all through the last few hours of labor. He kept me focused when my eyes would wander or close, by standing about one foot away from me while we breathed."

Praise your partner for the very hard work she's doing and keep encouraging her. One mother remembers, "Joe kept reminding me that we were progressing steadily. He was great for my morale. After each contraction he told me 'That was a beautiful contraction.' Corny as it sounds, that encouragement meant everything to me."

When she's pushing, keep telling her there's enough room for the baby to fit through (it won't feel that way to her!). It's especially important at this point to help her to stay "open" and to release the voluntary muscles around her vagina. She'll also need help to relax completely after each contraction in order to draw strength for the next one.

Helping a woman in labor is demanding work, but it's probably one of the most rewarding things you'll ever do. A new mother reflects back on her husband's help during her labor:

> He was able to relax me by focusing, eye contact, and verbal cues. He never gave up or tired of telling me what to do, or minded what I told him to do in my more unreasonable phases. I couldn't believe how much strength I drew from him and I know that I never could have managed without him. While I am usually very independent, I learned how to depend on him, both to keep me "together" during contractions, and to run interference for me with the hospital staff.

As Pat Summers said, "Birth was one of the peak experiences of my life. It became that because I had good support and we all worked together to make it so."

16
Setting the Mood:
The Birth Environment

When our cat was expecting her first litter of kittens, we researched the subject and compiled a cozy birthplace for her. A wicker basket lined with shredded newspapers and old scraps of cloth occupied a prominent spot in her favorite room, as we all waited expectantly for the big moment to arrive. When it did, the cat naturally ignored the designated basket. She chose instead to deliver her kittens on top of several layers of my daughter's clothes in an armoire.

Unless you're severely limited by geographical constraints, you, too, will be able to choose the birth environment that makes you most comfortable: traditional hospital delivery, in which you labor, deliver, and recover in separate rooms; labor-delivery-recovery room or birthing room in a hospital; out-of-hospital alternative birthing center; or home birth.

In the end, your comfort in the birthing environment of your choice will have a lot less to do with the way the place looks than with the way you're treated there. All the lovely wallpaper in the world can't make up for an unfriendly staff; but, fortunately, a supportive network of helpers can turn even the most unprepossessing environment into a fine place to have a baby.

Since the critical element in a good birth environment is the quality of the people who work there, pick your birth attendant and birth place carefully. Get recommendations from friends, and find out what they liked and didn't like about their births.

At least four out of five women giving birth in America go to obstetricians, physicians whose training encompasses birth as well as the surgical treatment of female reproductive problems. Another 15 percent or so go to family practitioners, medical doctors who are also qualified to treat other members of the family.

A small but growing number of women giving birth in the hospital choose the care of a certified nurse-midwife, a registered nurse who has undergone two additional years of training in midwifery. A certified nurse-midwife can take care of normal, healthy women through pregnancy, birth, and postpartum. In 1975 less than 1 percent of American women received their obstetrical care from a nurse-midwife, but in 1988 3.4 percent used nurse-midwives for hospital births.

If a nurse-midwife attends you for a hospital delivery, she will usually stay with you from the time you are admitted to the hospital until after your baby is born. One mother says, "I liked having a nurse-midwife for this delivery. It didn't feel so much like the assembly-room atmosphere at my first birth, where the obstetrician just ran in to catch the baby at the end."

If you are planning a home birth you may be cared for by either a doctor or a certified nurse-midwife. Or you might engage the services of a lay or "empirical" midwife. Sometimes called direct-entry midwives because they study midwifery without necessarily having gone through nursing training first, these women share with certified nurse-midwives a commitment to attend women throughout labor. But you should know that direct-entry midwives' training, licensure, and even legality vary from state to state. Two national organizations can give you current information on midwifery care for birth (see Resources).

When you first meet with a prospective birth attendant, try and bring your husband and be sure to ask about the issues that most concern both of you. You're looking for more than just "correct" answers to your questions. You want an attitude of respect, demonstrated by courtesy, sensible explanations, and a flexible attitude.

Even if you love your birth attendant, if the hospital is unpleasant, it's bound to affect your birth. Tour the hospital where your birth attendant practices to discover whether you'll be able to feel comfortable there. If you can, take two tours: one in early pregnancy while you still have time to change or negotiate hospital policies you don't like, and another later in pregnancy to get more information about labor and delivery procedures. Two of the most important things to determine on a tour are the type of support available from the nursing staff and how open the staff is to your bringing labor companions (see chapter 15).

Hospital Birth

Critics deride the American way of giving birth, but for some women a high-technology approach offers just the assurance they need to relax and let labor happen. Hospitals, of course, differ as to how much technology they routinely employ for birth (see chapter 17). This will depend also on your birth attendant's philosophy and on your particular needs during labor. Be sure to talk to your birth attendant about this and to take a hospital tour to learn just what routines and options are customarily offered. You could get some of this information by calling the head nurse of the maternity section.

In a traditional hospital delivery you would spend first-stage labor in a labor room, get wheeled to a delivery room for the birth, transfer to a recovery room for a brief period afterwards, and then stay in a postpartum room for a stay of one to three days. Recently, many hospitals have switched to a system of single-room maternity care in which a woman labors, delivers, recovers, and sometimes even recuperates in the same room (see LDRs and LDRPs, later in this chapter). Depending on your hospital, a cesarean may be performed in a regular delivery room or you may be moved to a surgical floor.

Although the effects of the environment on human labor haven't been well researched, environmental stresses have long been known to be disastrous to animal labor. In now-classic experiments, psychologist Niles Newton demonstrated that mice labored more quickly and lost significantly fewer of their offspring to stillbirth when they remained undisturbed during labor. Crowding, fear, noise, and being transferred from one place to another all caused animals to have more spontaneous abortions, stillbirths, and postpartum mothering failures.

Critics of American birth argue that human mothers in the hospital are also subject to the effects of a stressful labor environment. More than 40 years ago Grantly Dick-Read wrote, "Nothing is more irritating than noise and restlessness when relaxation is sought, or more exasperating than inconsequential chatter when the mind is occupied with an all-absorbing interest."

How the hospital environment affects you, of course, will depend on your own expectations and personality. Many women find that the hospital environment adds to their discomfort. One mother says, "There were three other women, all screaming their heads off. The combination of the phone ringing at the nurses' station, the bleep-bleep of the monitor, and the screaming women was enough to make me feel worse than ever."

Another mother found herself put off by the appearance of the labor room, "dreary and drab, painted in institutional gold. The ambience affected me immediately. The delivery room was another wretched-looking place. When the baby was born, his eyes peered all over and I wished that his first sight in the world had been something better than this uninspiring room."

But some women find hospitals reassuring. Suzanne Gordon, for example, appreciated her high-technology hospital delivery. She writes, "From the moment I entered its antiseptic corridors, donned the dreaded hospital johnny and strapped an ID band to my wrist, I felt at ease."

Especially if your birth attendants are supportive, you may well find the hospital environment a pleasant surprise. Recalling the intimate circle of people in the delivery room at his son's birth, a father says, "There was just the nurse who had stayed with us from admitting through delivery, the doctor, Judy, and I—a real personal experience. I'd expected a typical operating room, full of equipment, bright lights, and a generally impersonal atmosphere. However, the delivery room itself was simple and there were no bright lights except where they were needed. All in all, because of the staff, our hospital delivery was a truly joyful experience." As another mother puts it, "It's the people, not the place."

Unless you plan to be attended by a nurse-midwife, staff nurses are the people who will be working most closely with you during your labor. If you're going to a teaching hospital, you'll also be cared for by resident physicians until your own doctor arrives, usually toward the end of your labor.

At some hospitals, one-to-one nursing care is the standard. Rebecca Rosen-Horn, who worked as a labor and delivery nurse at Beth Israel Hospital in Boston for 11 years, says, "The whole hospital prides itself on its primary nursing. Because the patients get continuous labor support from one nurse, they need much less medication. By and large, we get rave reviews from laboring couples."

But, more often than not, labor and delivery nurses get assigned to more than one patient for the duration of their work shift. In addition to caring for you and her other patient(s), the nurse assigned to you has certain jobs that she must do—charting, checking fetal heart tones, giving medications, and following the doctor's orders. Linda Ungerleider, who teaches maternity nursing at North Park College in Chicago, explains why you might not see much of "your" labor nurse, especially if you and your partner seem well prepared for birth: "It can be a real conflict for a nurse if she has responsibility for two different women in labor, one of whom has no one with her while the other one has her husband." If you suspect your nurse might lack the time to offer you much consistent support, consider bringing a doula or monitrice with you in addition to your labor partner (see chapter 15).

Sometimes, how much nursing care you get depends not so much on how busy the hospital is but on how dedicated your nurse is to giving you support. Women are always grateful when they get a nurse who takes her helping role seriously. One such mother says, "My husband and the nurse who stayed with me throughout my labor were instrumental in helping me concentrate and continue with my breathing techniques. They were both wonderfully supportive, holding my hands, applying pressure to my back, giving me ice chips, and wiping me off with cold washcloths. Without the two of them I think I would have panicked and concentrated on the pain of the contractions rather than on the breathing and relaxing."

If you have decided about anything you particularly want or don't want during your labor, be sure you tell your nurse when you first are admitted to the hospital. Linda Ungerleider advises, "Let the nurse know: 'Some of my goals are. . . . ,' or 'If all goes well, we would like. . . .' Then the nurse can help you to achieve your goals."

One couple who shared their goal of avoiding medication for labor were pleased when their nurse supported them. According to the father, "The nurse said, 'If Carrie really needs medication, come and ask us. We won't offer it to her.' This simple statement made the whole labor progress better. Carrie and I knew we had to rely on our training and each other for support and help. And we did."

Many labor nurses will put their own preferences aside in order to support a woman's decisions about medication. Dinah Hobart, for example, has been a labor and delivery nurse for 25 years. She says, "Pain medication can add an element of dignity to someone who's out of control because of pain. I knew I wanted anesthesia as a part of my experience when I gave birth. I want parents to look at the experience as a pleasant one, but I try to support whatever the couple wants to do."

Some hospital staff members are less likely to be supportive if your ideas about birth are different from theirs. One mother told an obstetric resident that she'd like to avoid an epidural if possible. She says, "The resident laughed and said she didn't know why I would want to experience all that pain."

Even a woman who is highly motivated to avoid medication may find it hard to resist the hospital staff's offers of medication when she is actually in labor. Doctors and nurses sometimes suggest painkillers out of their own discomfort at seeing a woman in pain. Linda Ungerleider says, "It's a normal response for someone in the medical profession to want to relieve a person's pain." And the alternative is hard work, according to Ungerleider: "Watching a woman suffer, attempting to relieve back labor hour after hour."

In order to get the support you deserve, be sure you communicate your needs clearly and tactfully. Expect your birth attendants to be supportive, but if you're not getting help from the person who's been assigned to take care of you, tell the head nurse that you'd like a substitute caretaker. Dinah Hobart says, "It's so important to have trust in the people who are taking care of you."

In-Hospital Alternatives

By the end of the 1980s most hospitals with obstetric units had retooled their delivery services to offer some form of single-room care. According to American Hospital Association spokesperson Beril Basman, nearly three out of four respondents to a 1989 AHA survey had either supplemented or completely replaced their traditional delivery areas. Only 27 percent of the hospitals surveyed were still exclusively using the old-fashioned units in which a mother might be shuffled to four different rooms before she finally got sent home with her new baby.

Your own hospital may offer any or all of the following: birthing rooms, labor-delivery-recovery (LDR) or labor-delivery-recovery-postpartum (LDRP) rooms, or an alternative birthing center.

Birthing Rooms.   Birthing rooms were highly touted as a marketing device for hospitals in the late 1970s and early 1980s. Staffed by obstetricians, family practitioners, or certified nurse-midwives, such rooms were often nothing but fancy showcases, however. In many hospitals, the eligibility requirements for "low-risk" obstetrical patients disqualified almost every woman who sought to use the room. Staff members did not usually like the rooms, either, and many simply refused to deliver babies there.

If your own hospital has just one or two birthing rooms and the remaining rooms are the standard separate labor and delivery rooms, it may be difficult to qualify for the birthing room. Ask whether you can use the birthing room and whether you'll get wholehearted support from your birth attendants while you're there. The best way to judge your hospital's birthing room is not by looking at its physical attributes, but by assessing the attitudes of your birth attendant and the other personnel who staff it. Dr. Frederic Ettner, a family practitioner who does home deliveries and also attends births at St. Francis Hospital in Evanston, Illinois, says, "Patients shouldn't have to feel that the whole weaponry of the hospital will come down on them if one little thing goes wrong with their labor in the birthing room."

Ettner continues, "It really doesn't make a difference where a woman delivers; what makes a difference is this: are her attendants adhering to good obstetrical practice? Are they letting her move around and be in comfortable positions; are they offering appropriate suggestions and being supportive of what she's doing?"

If your hospital lacks single-room care, you might want to ask whether you can simply deliver in the labor room. This will help you avoid a rushed transfer to the delivery room at the last minute. As one mother put it, "It was so much easier and less awkward to be in a regular bed and not to be moved from one place to another in the middle of the process."

LDRs and LDRPs. As hospitals compete for obstetric patients, more and more of them are rebuilding their units to accommodate the new multiple-use rooms, LDRs and LDRPs. These rooms enable cost-conscious hospitals to make optimal use of both their space and their staff, who have been trained to care for a woman and her baby throughout their stay in the hospital.

Because all the equipment needed for a complicated delivery can be cunningly camouflaged in bureaus and closets, an LDR room might look something like your own bedroom or a nice motel room. But birth in a homey-looking LDR will not necessarily resemble a home delivery. In many LDRs and LDRPs, birth is assisted by all the machinery that hides in the closet on the hospital tour. This approach to birth may or may not appeal to you. Be sure to take a tour and talk to friends to see how supportive the medical staff will be of your individual needs and preferences when you give birth.

In-Hospital Birthing Centers. In the late 1970s and 1980s, in-hospital birthing centers provided an on-site alternative to women who sought to deliver with few or no interventions. Like birthing rooms, alternative birthing centers were almost always limited to low-risk women, and they enjoyed only a modest appeal among obstetricians and nurses. Now that most hospitals have provided single-room maternity care to all their obstetrical patients, regardless of risk, most in-hospital alternative birthing centers have closed.

What distinguished in-hospital birthing centers was not so much that they allowed birth to take place in one room. Instead, it was their low-technology approach to obstetrical intervention. A 1980 study of 500 births in a California birthing center, cited by Korte and Scaer in *A Good Birth, A Safe Birth*, revealed the safety of this low-technology alternative for low-risk mothers. A matched group of low-risk mothers delivering in the traditional delivery suites experienced many more complications of labor, including three times as many cesareans, and their babies suffered 15 times as many cases of fetal distress as did mother-baby pairs in the birthing center.

A different program proved that this low-technology approach could reap benefits, even in a group of very high-risk mothers. North Central Bronx Hospital, a New York City municipal hospital for the poor, serves a population in which seven out of ten mothers are considered high risk. One in nine mothers walks in to the hospital for the first time during labor. The staff—largely certified nurse-midwives—encourage the mothers to bring partners and to walk around during labor. The midwives rarely employ interventions such as electronic fetal monitoring, medications, and Pitocin. In 1988, according to an article in *Birth*, this approach resulted in a cesarean rate of 11.8 percent, less than half the national rate, and excellent maternal and fetal outcomes.

Alternative Birthing Centers (ABCs)

Out-of-hospital births are rare in this country. Just over one percent of births currently occur either in freestanding alternative birthing centers or at home. But the publicity surrounding these births has undoubtedly motivated many hospitals to liberalize their own birthing policies.

According to the National Association of Childbearing Centers, in late 1991 the United States had 135 functioning out-of-hospital alternative birthing centers. Fifty more ABCs were in various stages of development.

Usually staffed by certified nurse-midwives in collaboration with obstetricians and pediatricians, ABCs offer a homelike environment for birth. Alternative birthing centers contain basic medical equipment—IVs, fetal monitors, analgesics, oxygen, and incubators—but the ABC approach typically eschews the routine use of this technology.

Because stringent screening ensures that only low-risk women deliver in these centers, out-of-hospital birth centers can and do boast an enviable record of safety. In 1989 the *New England Journal of Medicine* published the results of a study of 11,814 women who were admitted to 84 different freestanding birthing centers. During labor, 15.8 percent of the women needed to be transferred to nearby hospitals. Maternal and fetal outcomes of the entire group compared very favorably to those of low-risk women delivering in hospitals and the cesarean rate was an astonishingly low 4.4 percent.

While critics argue that no out-of-hospital birth can ensure complete safety, birthing center advocates point to the fact that emergency transfers to the hospital happen very rarely. Of the women in the study just cited, only 2.4 percent needed to be transferred to the hospital for emergency reasons.

What a good freestanding birthing center has to offer is high-quality personalized and noninterventionist care at a much lower cost than the typical hospital delivery. In addition, since most mothers go home shortly after a birthing center birth, women can also save money on hospital postpartum room fees. Many freestanding birth centers (as well as birthing rooms in hospitals) include a home visit by a nurse practitioner or nurse-midwife in the basic fee.

Of course, if you're considering an out-of-hospital birthing center, you'll need to do some careful research. Visit the center, talk to other parents who have used it, and check with the National Association of Childbearing Centers (see Resources) to make sure the center is accredited. Qualifications will be slightly different at different centers, but generally you'll be discouraged from having an out-of-hospital birth if you: have a serious health problem such as heart disease or diabetes; are expecting twins; have a baby in a breech or transverse position; have had a serious problem in a previous pregnancy; or go into labor before 37 weeks or after 42 weeks of pregnancy.

Home Birth

No one is ever talked *into* a home birth. In fact, if you're planning to have your baby at home, many of your family and friends may already have tried to talk you out of it. Most obstetricians believe that no pregnancy can be considered sufficiently risk-free to warrant the possibility of a tragic emergency occurring in a home delivery.

The American College of Obstetricians and Gynecologists (ACOG) argues that home delivery is unsafe. "We are against it," says spokesperson Mort Lebow. "There are a certain percentage of births which are low-risk until they go into labor and delivery. In out-of-hospital births, the rate of transports hovers at around 20 percent. Most transfers are not life-threatening. But they can be and some are."

However, home birth advocates are fond of pointing out that hospitals have never been proven to be safer places than homes for low-risk women to give birth.

In fact, only one study has actually controlled every variable so that the backgrounds of the women in the hospital delivery group would be identical to the backgrounds of the women in the home delivery group. This study, by Dr. Lewis Mehl, found a much higher rate of complications in a group of 1,046 women delivering in the hospital than it did in the 1,046 women delivering at home. Mothers in the hospital group experienced significantly more inductions, forceps and cesarean deliveries, serious lacerations, and postpartum hemorrhages than did the home delivery mothers. In addition, their babies suffered more fetal distress, breathing problems at birth, neonatal infections, and birth injuries.

Home birth, of course, is not for everyone. A woman with any of the risk factors that rule out the use of an alternative birthing center (see page 181) should not give birth at home; nor is it a good idea if you can't find a well-trained and skilled birth attendant. You should be no further than a 15-minute ride from a hospital, and you'll have to arrange backup procedures with a doctor who has admitting privileges to this hospital in case you need to be transported during the course of your labor.

Because it's generally considered so risky to give birth at home, people will deem you responsible for any problems that occur, even if the problems are totally unrelated to the place of delivery. And, when you give birth at home, you do in fact have to take much more responsibility: you'll need to get the room organized, prepare your bed, and get things ready for the baby. With these limitations in mind, people who have had their babies at home usually agree that "there's no place like home" for birth.

That's because the hospital is unfamiliar territory for you. Psychologist Randi Ettner observes, "When you're in the hospital, you're dependent on the staff and dependent on your doctor—you *are* out of control. You learn in your childbirth classes that it's helpful to stand up and move around and change positions, and they come in and they put a fetal monitor on you and they tell you you can't move around. A lot of times you have the best intentions but once you're in the hospital, you really relinquish control."

In contrast, in your own home you have the "home court advantage." One mother says, "Now that we've had a home delivery, it would be very hard to go to the hospital for another delivery. At home you are absolutely free to handle your labor as you feel the need. I can't imagine a hospital that would have been receptive to as much moving around as I needed to do. The midwife came early and just stayed with me. She was very supportive and equally skilled.

"The thought of drugs or anesthesia never entered my mind during the entire birth process. Whenever I got discouraged or said that it hurt, someone was right there to tell me what a good job I was doing, to give me a drink, or to touch me. For me, loving care from people was a much better analgesic than drugs."

Toward an Ideal Birthing Environment

Dr. Michel Odent formerly directed the maternity unit at the hospital in Pithiviers, about 35 miles south of Paris. Under Odent's direction, Pithiviers became justly famous as a wonderful place to give birth. Odent specified that nothing at all in the birthing atmosphere should disrupt the mother's concentration on her fundamental task of giving birth. This translated into carte blanche for a mother to choose comfortable positions, to use warm baths for relaxation, and to walk as long as she felt comfortable doing so.

Although the clinic served women in every risk category, Pithiviers's mortality rate was enviably low. Their cesarean rate hovered around 7 percent, and their episiotomy rate was only 7.1 percent. Medication played no role in normal deliveries.

The environment Odent established at Pithiviers, right down to the color of the walls and curtains and the lack of any furniture to suggest a preferred posture, all contributed to a mother's ability to regress to a more instinctual level of behavior. Only at this level, Odent believes, can a mother give birth with ease.

In his introduction to Janet Balaskas's *Active Birth*, Odent describes what he considers to be the ideal environment for birth. The perfect birth environment, Odent writes, would ensure the mother "privacy, semi-darkness, silence, and, at the same time, the proximity of an experienced person." Odent now believes that only a woman's own home can provide such an environment. Since the majority of American women will probably continue to have their babies in the hospital, however, expectant parents must seek out a birthing environment where, as at Pithiviers, respect and support for the birthing family inform every administrative decision.

17

Hospital Routines:
Is the Gain
Worth the Pain?

When you're pregnant, you want to do what's best for your baby's welfare. Unfortunately, experts disagree on exactly what that means, especially when it comes to applying technology to the birth process. Technologies that can be lifesaving for high-risk childbirth— IVs, Pitocin, and electronic fetal monitoring, for example—often get used for deliveries where they are not needed. Critics contend that this turns normal birth into a pathological event in which an expectant woman is treated as a high-risk patient until she can prove herself otherwise. And, she can do so only *after* her baby is born.

Each form of intervention carries certain risks. These are worth taking in high-risk situations where the potential benefits appear to outweigh the drawbacks. But in low-risk situations, technological interventions usually offer no advantages. They only add risk and discomfort without providing any compensatory benefits.

Not only can unnecessary interventions be painful in themselves. They may also raise your anxiety level, prompting a catecholamine surge that will reduce your uterine efficiency and contribute further to the length and discomfort of your labor. Several years ago, author and childbirth educator Penny Simkin surveyed 159 of her students who had recently experienced vaginal births. Simkin asked the new mothers which interventions they found stressful. At least half of her sample rated each of the following birth interventions moderately or very stressful:

- Pitocin induction or augmentation of labor.
- Electronic fetal monitoring.
- Vaginal examinations during labor.
- Intravenous fluids (IVs).
- Analgesia or anesthesia.
- Restriction to bed or restriction of movement in bed.
- Restriction of fluids.
- Unfamiliar or less preferred doctor.
- Episiotomy.
- Forceps or vacuum extractor.
- Limitations of time with the baby.
- Circumcision.

Since many of these interventions can be avoided or have legitimate alternatives, do a bit of advance planning. First, consider which procedures might raise your own stress level. Then learn which procedures are mandatory or advisable and which may be superfluous in your particular case. With this information, you'll be better able to participate with your birth attendant in making informed decisions about the appropriate use of technology during your labor.

Of course you have the right to refuse any interventions during your birth. But it's much better to communicate openly before labor begins so you and your birth attendant can discover whether you're in basic agreement about the way you'd like the birth to go. Because childbirth can't be scripted, you'll need to make your game plan a flexible one. Still, it's important to express your preferences and for you to understand what your birth attendant expects, too.

Where you give birth makes a big difference. Home deliveries, and births in birthing rooms and alternative birthing centers, tend to be very individualized events (see chapter 16). But even traditional hospital deliveries can be tailored to your preferences if you express them clearly. If you're giving birth in the hospital and learn that a particular item is a "hospital routine," remember that it's doctors who make hospital policy. Discuss with your doctor any routines you feel are objectionable before you go into labor, and see whether an exception can be made in your case.

A Shave and an Enema: Vestiges of a Bygone Era.   Two rituals that have almost disappeared from today's childbirth scene are the shave and the enema. Formerly a woman's pubic hair got shaved for two reasons: to prevent infection and to keep hair out of the episiotomy site. The shave itself often hurt and the pubic hair itched as it grew back. Worst of all, research showed that not only did shaving not prevent infection, it actually *increased* the rate of infection because of tiny nicks from the razor. If you are going to have an episiotomy, you may need just a very minimal clip or shave of the hairs right on your perineum. Many women don't need even this.

In the 300 years it has played a role in obstetric practice, the enema has had three major benefits claimed for it. First, an enema stimulates uterine activity; second, it makes room for the descent of the baby's head; third, and most important, it reduces contamination of the delivery area.

But taking an enema does not always shorten labor or keep the delivery area clean. In 1981, a British study randomly assigned laboring women to an enema or a non-enema group. The researchers found that the enema made no difference in the length of labor or in whether or not the women passed stool during birth. At first, the midwives who conducted the trial were reluctant to participate because they believed so firmly in the benefits of routine enemas. Ironically, the study had to be called off early because when the midwives saw that enemas made no difference, they refused to give them to the women who had been randomly assigned to the enema group!

Because most women get frequent loose bowel movements before they go into labor, an enema may be superfluous for you. But you may choose to give yourself an enema at home or get one in the hospital if you have been eating normally and haven't moved your bowels for at least a day before labor begins. Or you may want to use an enema or castor oil to stimulate contractions in early labor (see Pitocin, page 192).

Some women simply don't feel completely comfortable about pushing in the second stage of labor if they're worried that they may expel stool as they push. Request an enema if you think it will make your labor more comfortable, but bear in mind that the period of time it takes to expel the enema—about 20 to 30 minutes—will probably be accompanied by stronger, more painful uterine contractions.

For years, women found the enema a demeaning and uncomfortable part of giving birth. Now, in most hospitals, an enema is an option, not a routine. One labor and delivery nurse says, "If you want an enema in our labor room nowadays, you have to ask for one."

Intravenous Line (IV). You may get an intravenous line to give you fluids or to keep a vein open in case you need emergency medications. Of course, you probably won't need an IV for fluids if you will be able to drink water, tea, or juice throughout labor. But you certainly will get an IV if you receive narcotic painkillers or a regional anesthetic such as an epidural block. The epidural, in particular, tends to lower your blood pressure, and IV fluids can help to maintain it at a healthy level. Since Pitocin can be given most safely by vein, its administration also mandates the use of an IV. You will probably also require intravenous fluids if you show an abnormal labor pattern, excessive vomiting, or signs of dehydration or exhaustion.

An IV can be helpful if you need it. But critics like psychologist Niles Newton point out that the routine use of an IV heightens your risk for problems such as inflammation, infection, fluid overdose, and even pulmonary embolism. Not only do IV fluids provide inadequate nutrition for the strenuous process of labor, their prolonged use in labor may cause electrolyte or blood sugar imbalance. Electrolytes are blood chemicals responsible for maintaining a normal fluid balance in your body. An imbalance in your own blood sugar during labor can cause a rebound hypoglycemia (low blood sugar) in your infant.

Probably the most pervasive complaint about the IV is that it changes your image of yourself—once you're on the IV, you're no longer a healthy woman going through a normal process, but a patient. Joanne Slavin, associate professor of nutrition at the University of Minnesota, observes, "Being hooked up to an IV makes you into a sick person. It's not something a well person would want to do." The IV certainly can make it more challenging to move and change positions during labor. If you are permitted to walk, you can get an IV on a pole with wheels, but you will no longer be "traveling light."

It may also be painful when the IV needle is inserted, particularly if the person doing the insertion has little experience. One mother recalls, "Our labor nurse was wonderful in all respects, but she couldn't put in an IV. After trying in both arms and causing me much pain, she called for the IV nurse who got the needle in with one shot." Finally, the fluid from the IV may leak into the tissues outside of your vein, leading to some local tenderness.

In addition to questioning whether routine IVs are needed to give women fluids in labor, many experts also question whether an IV must be inserted to keep a vein open for an emergency. They make three arguments. First, it's unlikely that your veins will collapse quickly, even in an emergency. Second, if your veins do collapse, a minor surgical procedure called a "cut-down" can be performed quickly to get medication into your bloodstream. Finally, if your vein must be left open, a "heparin lock" can be put into place instead of an IV. The tiny heparin lock leaves your vein open but doesn't require attaching you to the whole IV apparatus.

At some hospitals, IVs are mandatory from the start of labor, while at other hospitals, IVs are reserved for women whose labors are high-risk. Even if your doctor prefers to have his or her patients use an IV routinely, you may be able to negotiate for the use of an IV on an as-needed basis, or to get the more portable heparin lock. If you get an IV, ask to have an experienced staff person insert it into the hand you use least.

Electronic Fetal Monitoring.   The fetal monitor simultaneously assesses your baby's heartbeat and your contractions in order to give continuous information about how your baby is responding to the stress of labor. About the size of a video cassette recorder, the machine sits atop a table next to your bed in the labor room. Information about your contractions and your baby's heartbeat feeds continuously out of the front of the machine onto a long strip of graph paper.

The electronic fetal monitor allows you to see your contractions as they are happening and also to "see" your baby's heart beating along at a healthy clip of about 120 to 160 beats per minute. A volume control on the machine allows you to hear the heartbeat, too, if you want to. It sounds something like a horse galloping under water.

Fetal monitoring can be done externally or internally, depending on your particular situation and your doctor's preference. External monitoring employs two elastic belts around your abdomen. The top belt has a pressure-sensitive gauge which reacts to the changing shape of your abdomen as your uterus alternately contracts and relaxes. Since the contraction begins at the fundus, or top, of the uterus, but you can't feel it until it reaches the cervix a few seconds later, many women use the fetal monitor printout to cue their relaxation and breathing at the very beginning of each contraction.

The second belt, worn closer to your groin, has an ultrasound device which "hears" your baby's heart valves opening and closing, and transmits this signal to the machine where it translates into a numerical representation of beats per minute. External monitoring is subject to movement artifact, which means that when you or your baby moves, the numbers may be thrown off. Even if the belt for the baby's heartbeat is constantly readjusted—and it may need to be—the heart rate registered by the ultrasound device in the monitor is not 100 percent accurate. If a serious question arises about your baby's condition, internal monitoring will probably be substituted.

Internal monitoring requires that your amniotic sac be ruptured (see Amniotomy, page 192) and that you be at least two or three centimeters dilated. The baby's heartbeat will be monitored internally by means of a tiny spiral electrode. This is inserted through a slender tube up your vagina and cervix; the tip is then nudged about a millimeter or two under your baby's scalp. The internal electrode provides a completely accurate EKG (electrocardiogram) reading.

Your contractions could also be monitored internally by the insertion of a tiny catheter into your uterus, or you could have a combination of external and internal monitoring, the baby being monitored internally while you retain the contraction-monitoring belt around your abdomen.

Your baby will probably show a healthy heartbeat. But if your baby's heartbeat indicates fetal distress, you may be asked to turn onto your side, be given oxygen, or have your Pitocin drip turned off. If your baby fails to perk up with these measures, a rapid delivery by forceps or cesarean may be necessary. Some doctors will further corroborate a diagnosis of fetal distress before rushing to do an emergency cesarean. They may stimulate the baby with pressure or sound, checking to see if one of these stimulants jogs the baby's heartbeat into a normal rise. Or they may take a tiny sample of the baby's scalp blood to check for acidity. These interventions can prevent an unnecessary cesarean for fetal distress (see Cesarean Birth, page 199).

Receiving constant information about your baby's well-being can be very reassuring to expectant parents, and you may find the rhythmic sounds of your baby's heartbeat soothing "music to your ears." Seeing the contractions before you can feel them may also be very helpful to you as a form of biofeedback (see chapter 12). In addition, electronic fetal monitoring can be an advantage to your labor if you're in a high-risk situation. It's considered mandatory if you receive medication or if your labor is induced or augmented with Pitocin (see Pitocin, page 192).

But being monitored electronically has its drawbacks. One mother wrote, in a letter to *Parents* magazine: "The biggest difference the laboring mother experiences is that with fetal monitoring, she *can't* move. . . . A second difference is that without fetal monitoring, continuous attention by the birth attendant becomes a necessity, because she or he must continually listen for the baby's heartbeat with a stethoscope. This provides a continuity of service to the laboring woman that is extremely reassuring."

Being monitored continuously certainly hampers your mobility in labor. You can change positions in bed or move to a chair, but you are on a very short tether. Furthermore, the belts can be uncomfortably tight and they usually need to be adjusted when you do move. Many women accommodate by spending their labors lying rigidly in one position for the supposed benefit of the machine and the hospital staff, but to their own great discomfort and perhaps to the detriment of their babies. If you lie on your back to be monitored, for example, you could actually be creating the very fetal distress the fetal monitor is supposed to detect (see page 202).

Despite the widespread use of the electronic fetal monitor, eight studies have failed to demonstrate that babies who are monitored electronically throughout labor fare better than babies whose heartbeats are auscultated (listened to) by trained nurses. Summarizing these studies in 1988, the Executive Board of the American College of Obstetricians and Gynecologists (ACOG) concluded that not only did routine electronic fetal monitoring show no benefit over manual auscultation, it had also led to a significant rise in cesarean deliveries. ACOG concluded that auscultation was as effective as electronic fetal monitoring for low-risk mothers.

But auscultation with a hand-held stethoscope or the Doppler, a portable ultrasound device, requires almost constant nursing attendance. So this option may be unavailable unless your hospital offers one-to-one nursing care, or you are being attended by a nurse-midwife or your own monitrice (see chapter 15).

In light of ACOG's recommendations, many laboring mothers today get monitored electronically on an intermittent basis, usually about 15 minutes out of each hour. You might also ask if your hospital offers radio telemetry, which continuously monitors your baby's heart rate by ultrasound, but also allows you to be mobile. As you walk around, a wireless transmitter (telemetry unit) clipped to your gown radios your baby's heart rate back to your room or to the nurses' station. A small study compared two groups of women, one of which was monitored by radio telemetry and the other of which got routine monitoring. Perhaps because they could move around freely throughout labor, the telemetry group used much less anesthesia than did the mothers who were confined to bed by the standard monitoring system.

If you prefer not to be monitored continuously throughout your labor, discuss your desires with your birth attendant and plan in advance to be auscultated by your nurse, nurse-midwife, or monitrice; to be monitored intermittently; or to use radio telemetry monitoring.

Since you may well be electronically monitored for at least part of your labor, ask your nurse to show you how to readjust the belts so you can move more freely without losing the baby's heartbeat. You may also want to ask for some talcum powder to put under the belts so that they feel more comfortable around your abdomen.

Amniotomy.   Your bag of waters could break naturally at any time before or during labor, but most likely will stay intact until you begin pushing at the start of second stage. Or, your doctor might break your bag in a procedure called amniotomy. Amniotomy ("snagging the bag" is what they call it in the hospital) gets performed with an instrument that looks like a long plastic crochet hook.

A British study found that the advantages of routine amniotomy— the ability to examine the amniotic fluid and the capacity to do internal fetal monitoring—outweighed the risks. In this study, amniotomy shortened labor by an average of more than two hours and reduced the need for both Pitocin augmentation and forceps delivery. Babies whose mothers had amniotomies and those whose mothers did not showed no differences in Apgar scores, blood acidity, jaundice, or admissions to neonatal intensive-care units.

Some mothers appreciate having their bag of waters artificially broken. A second-time mother says, "The doctor broke my bag of waters when I was dilated to nine centimeters. It was the nicest thing anybody ever did for me. What relief! The nurse said it had been the bag of waters causing all the rectal pressure. Once it was done, I was dilated to ten almost immediately and they started getting the bed and me ready for delivery."

Amniotomy itself is painless, though the contractions frequently become a great deal stronger and you're likely to be confined to bed after your membranes are ruptured. One mother says, "The doctor decided to break my water bag. This sent me into transition immediately. I wasn't prepared for the sudden change. The first contraction was severe and caught me off guard. The pain in my back became unbearable."

Critics of artificial rupture contend that the fluid in the amniotic sac provides an important cushion for your baby's head, preventing excessive molding of the baby's skull bones and compression of his umbilical cord. In addition, amniotomy with the baby in a breech position or when the baby's head is high can risk umbilical cord prolapse. According to some studies, amniotomy rarely speeds labor by more than about 30 to 40 minutes, so you may prefer to allow nature to take its own course. You should also know that once your bag is broken, delivery must necessarily take place within a maximum of 24 hours, in order to prevent infection. Therefore, amniotomy may necessitate the use of Pitocin.

Pitocin.   Labor normally begins around your due date. At that time, signals received from your baby and your body stimulate the pituitary gland to release oxytocin, a hormone that causes uterine contractions. At times it's necessary to give this natural process a nudge, either to begin it or to boost labor should it falter.

A woman with confirmed postmaturity, active herpes without lesions at term, diabetes, hypertension, Rh problems, or prolonged premature rupture of the membranes may be a candidate for induction, either for her own health or for the welfare of her baby.

If you get Pitocin—synthetic oxytocin—it will be given through your IV in carefully-controlled increments. An induced or augmented labor must be scrupulously monitored because if the dosage is too high, your uterus may go into a tetanic contraction, reducing blood flow through the placenta and putting your baby in jeopardy. The use of Pitocin may also "telescope" labor, making it difficult to cope without painkillers.

A study published recently in *Obstetrics and Gynecology* suggested that a slowly accelerating low-dose regimen of Pitocin mimics the normal physiologic course of labor much more closely than does the standard regimen. Though it took longer for the low dose to bring on active labor, women in the low-dose group experienced fewer abnormal fetal heart rates and far fewer cesareans.

In the past, Pitocin was used quite frequently for "elective induction," so-called because medical indications for immediate birth were lacking or questionable. But Pitocin can render uterine contractions stronger and more frequent, depriving a baby at risk of the normal recovery time "to catch his breath" between contractions. Today, the Food and Drug Administration (FDA) mandates that Pitocin be used only when induction is medically necessary for the safety of mother or baby.

But medical necessity isn't always clear-cut. One of the most debated questions in obstetrics is this: How many hours may pass after a premature rupture of the membranes before a woman and her baby are considered at risk for infection and appropriate candidates for a Pitocin induction? In recent years, the number of hours has been progressively reduced. But some experts contend that membrane rupture by itself does not necessarily increase the incidence of infection. What seems to contribute more to an increased rate of infection is the timing of the first vaginal exam after the bag of waters is broken.

In a study published in *Obstetrics and Gynecology* in 1989, a group of women with ruptured membranes were left for 24 hours to see if they would begin labor on their own. Three-fourths of the women did. Eighteen women with ruptured membranes received initial vaginal exams, while 78 women did not. Five infants in the examined group got infections. Not one of the infants in the groups without exams got infected.

Two older studies, one from Great Britain and one from Texas, also showed that when women with ruptured membranes received no vaginal exams but were allowed to await spontaneous labor, the vast majority began labor on their own within 24 hours. What's more, they didn't incur any more infections than did the induced groups, and they had shorter labors and far fewer cesareans.

You may want to discuss with your birth attendant what course you should follow if your bag of waters breaks before you go into labor. Some birth attendants will encourage you to wait at home, perhaps taking your temperature to be sure you aren't developing a fever. Others may require you to come to the hospital to be checked, perhaps with a sterile speculum rather than a gloved hand. In general, once your bag of waters is broken, the fewer internal examinations the better.

Though it still lacks the approval of the FDA, prostaglandin gel is used widely in Europe and at many medical centers in the United States to ripen the cervix of a woman who would otherwise be a candidate for induction. This outpatient treatment appears to reduce the need for Pitocin. Prostaglandin gel has also been shown to reduce induction failures, thereby lowering the rate of cesareans for failure to progress. But you should be aware that this treatment can occasionally cause nausea, blood pressure changes, or extremely strong contractions.

Several other alternatives to Pitocin exist. Bathing, walking, and TENS stimulation of acupuncture points have all been discussed in previous chapters. Sexual or nipple stimulation are also related to natural oxytocin release, although if your bag of waters is broken, you shouldn't insert anything into your vagina. You may want to begin to stimulate your nipples at around 38 or 39 weeks in order to "ripen" your cervix and minimize your chances of needing to be induced, should you go too far past your due date. Be careful, though, not to hyperstimulate your uterus. It's best to gently stimulate one nipple at a time, and to stop if you get a contraction that lasts 45 seconds or longer.

You may also use nipple stimulation to promote labor once it has begun. One mother who used nipple stimulation during labor reports, "It hurt when Ken stimulated my nipples, but it made my contractions stronger and that was what we needed."

Bowel stimulation is another way to get labor started or to intensify it. If you prefer to avoid an enema, you might try at half-hour intervals two to four tablespoons of castor oil mixed with orange juice. But don't take this mixture more than three times.

The patience and sensitivity of your birth attendant or labor partner occasionally can avert the need for Pitocin. Dr. Mitchell Levine, an obstetrician in Cambridge, Massachusetts, suggests that you consider what may be holding you back if your labor is prolonged. He says, "Old, unresolved issues can stop labor. It's amazing how sensitive the body and labor are to anger, fear, and other kinds of emotional concerns. Sometimes talking about these issues beforehand makes all the difference."

Episiotomy. This common surgical procedure enlarges the vaginal opening just before birth. Depending on your birth attendant, if you're having your first baby, your chances of having an episiotomy could be as high as 90 percent.

Episiotomy has its place in medical practice. The cut can speed delivery by a few minutes, a margin of speed that may make a difference to a baby in distress. It can help a baby through a tight and unyielding perineum, or reduce pressure on the head of a fragile premie. Episiotomy can also facilitate the application of forceps or vacuum extractor (see later).

First described in the medical literature in 1742, episiotomy has been claimed to have four major benefits:

- A clean cut is easier to repair and heals better than a spontaneous laceration.
- Episiotomy prevents serious lacerations into the anus.
- Episiotomy spares the baby's head a lengthy pushing stint, which might lead to brain injury.
- Episiotomy prevents future damage to a woman's pelvic floor muscles.

But a survey of the medical literature on episiotomy by Drs. David Banta and Stephen B. Thacker revealed no evidence that episiotomy actually produced any of the benefits listed above. On the other hand, Banta and Thacker found the obstetrical literature replete with documentation on the procedure's risks: 60 percent of the women who underwent episiotomy experienced severe pain, and 20 percent experienced problems with intercourse for up to three months after delivery. Swelling was common and wound infections occurred in one to four women out of a hundred. Two studies subsequently published in the *British Medical Journal* revealed no evidence that reducing the episiotomy rate prolonged the second stage, traumatized babies' heads, or did long-term damage to mothers' pelvic floor muscles.

There are two types of episiotomy: the midline, which prevails in the United States, and the mediolateral, which is more common in Great Britain. The midline cut goes straight down toward the anus and approximates the direction of a tear that might occur naturally. This cut is less painful, heals more quickly, and produces less blood loss than does a mediolateral incision, which angles on the bias.

But a midline episiotomy is also more likely than a mediolateral cut to extend into the anus. It is also much more likely to do so than is a natural tear. A clinical study that appeared in *Obstetrics and Gynecology* in 1987 compared a group of women who received routine midline episiotomies with a control group, on whom episiotomies were performed only if medically warranted. The researchers found that *only* women who had been given episiotomies suffered lacerations into the anus. So instead of preventing tears, routine midline episiotomies appeared to initiate them. In recent years, a spate of other research papers published in the *American Journal of Obstetrics and Gynecology* and *Obstetrics and Gynecology* have supported this finding. It's easy to understand why episiotomies may extend into tears if you think for a moment about how you make an old sheet into rags. It's difficult to tear the sheet until you cut it. But as soon as you make a snip, the sheet tears easily.

Nancy Fleming, Ph.D., a certified nurse-midwife and clinical director of the Comprehensive Women's Health Care Center in Hinsdale, Illinois, wrote her doctoral dissertation on episiotomy. In Fleming's study, even women who required stitches for a natural tear seemed to fare at least as well as, if not better than, the women who received episiotomies. Here's why:

Birth tears are graded according to their severity. A first-degree laceration tears only skin, a second-degree laceration involves the underlying muscle, a third-degree laceration extends to the anus, and a fourth-degree laceration goes into the rectum. Many women who deliver without episiotomy don't tear at all. Or, they may sustain tiny first-degree tears that don't need stitches. Others get tears that range from minimal to moderate. But *every* woman who receives an episiotomy suffers at least a second-degree laceration, and a fair number of these cuts extend into serious third- and fourth-degree tears.

Probably the best way to avoid an unnecessary episiotomy is to choose your birth attendant carefully and express your preference clearly. If your doctor says, "I only do an episiotomy when it's necessary," see if you can get him or her to be more specific about when it might be necessary and what he might recommend to help you avoid it. If coached properly on restraining their pushing efforts, most women can deliver their babies over an intact perineum or with minor tears. Many writers have suggested that these naturally occurring tears heal more comfortably than does an episiotomy.

Obstetricians tend to perform episiotomy more than midwives, but many doctors are trying to meet their patients' desires to give birth with less intervention. Just be sure to reach agreement on this subject *before* you go into labor. When you're giving birth is a very difficult time to question your birth attendant's medical judgment that an episiotomy needs to be done.

One mother told her doctor she'd prefer not to have an episiotomy for her first birth. The baby weighed nine pounds, and she says, "Dr. Edwards stretched my perineum with his finger as the baby crowned so that no episiotomy was needed. The stretching was painful. But I'm glad not to have the stitches now."

Another mother compares her second birth—without an episiotomy—to her first:

> Having had a baby with and without episiotomy, I can say without reservation that without is better! It is now two days post-delivery and my bottom is only slightly sore. I have no problems with sitting, walking, any movements at all. While the doctor's manipulation of the vaginal opening to stretch it made me sore—somewhat like continually rubbing your tongue on an irritation in your mouth—it was minor compared with the extended postpartum discomfort of an episiotomy. The two small lacerations I experienced must have been very small since my only awareness of them is occasional burning on urination, much like getting salty water on a wound. I rarely feel even this. I really feel very good.

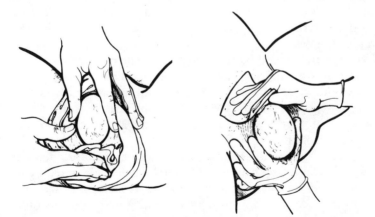

A warm compress (left), *can relax your perineum, reducing the need for an episiotomy and minimizing the likelihood of a tear. Right, the birth attendant allows the baby's head to ease out slowly.*

Doing the following things during labor will help you avoid tearing: Get into a good, gravity-enhancing position for pushing. Don't
spread your legs too far apart, because that puts extra stress on your
perineum. Relax your pelvic floor muscles, and allow your baby's
head to be born slowly. If you have had an epidural for pain relief in
labor, let it wear off before you begin pushing. Ask your birth attendants to use warm compresses or oil to permit your perineum to
stretch without tearing. And you may also want to prepare yourself
beforehand with perineal massage (see chapter 8).

Forceps.   These metal instruments to aid a vaginal delivery look
something like giant salad tongs. Forceps have two parts—branches—that lock at the intersection so that the blades cannot squeeze
your baby's head. The blades are not sharp and are designed with
curves to conform to your vagina and your baby's head.

Forceps may be used in the second (pushing) stage of labor if the
birth needs to be hastened, if your baby's head is too big or in the
wrong position to be born without assistance, or if you are unable to
continue pushing.

An instrumental delivery is termed "high forceps" if the baby's
head isn't yet engaged in the mother's pelvis, "midforceps" if the
baby's head is engaged but not visible, "low forceps" if the head is
visible at the vaginal opening, and "outlet forceps" if the head is dis-
tending the perineum. The higher forceps are used, the greater is the
potential risk to both baby and mother. High-forceps deliveries—significantly associated with trauma to the baby's head, shoulders, and
arms—have virtually disappeared because they proved much riskier
than cesarean delivery.

If you get an epidural block during labor, you're much more likely
to need a forceps delivery, for two reasons. First, epidural block
reduces both your urge to push and your sensation of pushing.
Second, an epidural relaxes your pelvic floor muscles, sometimes to
the extent that your baby's head fails to rotate and therefore requires
a midforceps rotation.

Babies delivered by forceps may show facial bruises for a few days
or may not exhibit any marks at all. Rarely, a baby delivered by forceps will suffer an intracranial hemorrhage or nerve damage to his
face and arms. As with any obstetric intervention, the benefits of forceps use should outweigh the risks.

Mothers who are delivered by forceps usually get a larger episiotomy. Even with an episiotomy, however, you're at greater risk for cervical and perineal tears if your delivery is accomplished with forceps.

In Europe and at some medical centers in this country a promising alternative to forceps has emerged. This alternative, the vacuum extractor, consists of a cap applied to the top of the baby's head and connected to a vacuum pump that supplies suction pressure. When the doctor pulls on the cap, the baby's head moves down.

The soft plastic or rubber cap has been determined to be as safe as forceps for the baby, although he may be born with a temporary swelling on his scalp at the application site. Several studies have confirmed that, compared to forceps, the vacuum extractor means fewer lacerations, less pain, and less blood loss for mothers who need assistance with their deliveries.

Cesarean Birth

In 1990, 23.5 percent of American women gave birth to their babies by cesarean section. Cesarean birth can be a life-saving operation and it's certainly become a much safer operation than it used to be. But you should bear in mind that every type of surgery has its risks and cesarean birth is no exception.

In comparison to vaginal birth, cesarean birth exposes you to several potential dangers. These include two to four times the risk of maternal death (primarily associated with general anesthesia) and five to ten times the risk of postpartum infection. In addition, recovering from a cesarean usually takes much longer than does recovery from a vaginal birth.

In his book *The Cesarean Myth*, Dr. Mortimer Rosen says that many people accept our current high cesarean rate because they believe in several myths about this method of delivery. According to Rosen, the following are commonly believed *myths*, not truths, about cesarean birth: 1) Cesareans are safe; 2) Cesareans are necessary in a broad range of cases; and 3) Cesareans produce healthier babies.

Because the quadrupling of our country's cesarean rate from 5.5 percent in 1970 has not led to a significant improvement in neonatal outcome, a fair amount of public criticism has accompanied the steep rise in cesareans. In 1989 the Public Citizen Health Research Group published a booklet entitled *Unnecessary Cesarean Sections: How to Cure a National Epidemic*. The authors, Dr. Lynn Silver and Dr. Sidney M. Wolfe, contended that at least 50 percent of the cesareans performed in the United States were unnecessary.

When *is* a cesarean necessary? You'll need a cesarean if your baby's head is too large for your pelvis, or if he is in distress that can't be reversed; if your baby is in a position that would prevent a safe vaginal delivery; if your baby's umbilical cord is coming first through the vagina; if your labor fails to progress sufficiently for a vaginal delivery; if the placenta blocks your cervix or detaches early; or if you have a disease which would pose dangers for you or your baby in the case of a vaginal delivery. Any of these circumstances would render a cesarean delivery the best alternative.

But why are you so much more likely than your mother was to have a cesarean? A litigious medicolegal climate that makes doctors more likely to intervene in the birth process, changes in obstetric fashion that now dictate cesareans for breeches and other risky births, and more deliveries of women with medical conditions that necessitate cesarean birth—all have contributed to the rise in cesareans.

Most cesareans today get performed for one of the following four indications: previous cesarean section; failure to progress in labor; fetal distress; and breech presentation. In fact, however, none of these four indications should routinely dictate a surgical delivery.

Previous cesarean section.   Of the 957,000 cesareans performed in 1989, 35.6 percent were routine repeat cesareans, despite ACOG's 1988 recommendation of vaginal birth after cesarean (VBAC) for almost every woman with a previous cesarean. When ACOG surveyed more than 2,000 obstetricians in 1990, nine out of ten doctors said they currently offer the option of VBAC to their patients. But ACOG spokesman Mort Lebow added, "We don't know how they're offering it." Subtle or overt encouragement to have a repeat cesarean—a faster, more lucrative, and easier delivery for the doctor—may account for the fact that in 1990 only 20.4 percent of women with previous cesareans had VBACs.

But the number of women having VBACs should ideally approach three out of four, according to Dr. Bruce Flamm, assistant clinical professor of obstetrics and gynecology at the University of California at Irvine and author of *Birth after Cesarean.*

If you've had a previous cesarean and would like to have a VBAC, take time to research your hospital and birth attendant. Ask for their cesarean and VBAC rates. If you're told that your hospital can't do VBACs because it's unequipped to do an emergency cesarean for uterine rupture (an extremely rare, but frequently innocuous risk of VBAC—most "ruptures" are actually asymptomatic thinnings of the uterine scar), look for another place to give birth. Several other obstetric emergencies, including cord prolapse and abrupted placenta, are at least as common as uterine rupture; these emergencies can occur whether or not a woman has had a previous cesarean. Dr. Flamm puts it bluntly: "Any hospital that is not prepared to allow VBAC should not be doing obstetrics."

Failure to Progress in Labor.   About one cesarean in three is performed for this "catch-all" category, which includes cephalopelvic disproportion and very long labors. Of mothers having their first babies, failure to progress is by far the most common cause of cesarean delivery. Any method that promotes the natural process of labor, but particularly remaining upright and active as long as possible (see chapter 10), should help you avoid having an unnecessary cesarean for this indication.

Breech.   About 15 percent of cesareans are performed because the baby is in a bottom-first or breech position. Because breech birth poses risks for an infant, many doctors advocate routine cesareans for all breech babies. Indeed, by 1989 almost 84 percent of breech babies were delivered surgically, compared to only about 10 percent in 1970. But routinely delivering all breech babies by cesarean cannot always guarantee a safe delivery. Accordingly, many doctors believe it makes more sense to try and turn a breech baby to a safer, head-down position.

A baby who is breech between 32 and 36 weeks will likely turn on his own; about nine out of ten do. To maximize your breech baby's chances of turning, you might try one of these two positions:

> Assume a knee-chest position—head and arms on a pillow, knees on the floor, and bottom in the air—for 15 minutes every two hours while you're awake.

> Lie on your back, knees bent and feet flat on the floor, with your hips raised by pillows to a height of 12 inches. Try this several times a day for ten or 15 minutes, but not immediately after a meal.

You may also try to lure your baby into a head-down position by playing music where you want your baby's head to be. Place a tape recorder or stereo headphones by your pubic bone, and experiment with different types of music to see if the "Pied Piper" approach works.

If your baby remains breech at 36 or 37 weeks, ask your doctor about external cephalic version, a medical procedure in which the doctor gently guides a breech baby from the outside. In numerous studies version has boasted a success rate of 60 to 70 percent in turning breech babies. The procedure does carry some risk of disturbing the placenta or compressing the baby's cord. But with appropriate safeguards external version may help you avoid the risks of breech birth for your baby and the risks of surgery for you. Alternately, you could choose to consult an acupuncturist to try and turn your breech baby (see chapter 7).

A breech baby may also be delivered vaginally by an experienced and open-minded birth attendant. You should ask your birth attendant if your breech baby is in a safe position for trying this alternative. Then discuss the risks and benefits of a vaginal breech birth.

Fetal Distress.   Ten percent of cesareans are performed to expedite the delivery of a baby whose heartbeat shows changes that don't respond when Pitocin is turned off, when the mother gets fluids or oxygen, or when she changes her position. But not every baby whose heart rate dips is actually suffering from fetal distress. In fact, according to Diony Young and Dr. Charles Mahan in their booklet *Unnecessary Cesareans: Ways to Avoid Them*, "If physicians relied exclusively on the electronic fetal monitor to decide whether to perform a cesarean, three women would have unnecessary cesareans for every one infant with real fetal distress." (See Electronic Fetal Monitoring, page 189).

Young and Mahan suggest several ways to try to avoid a needless cesarean. They recommend: picking your birth attendant and birthplace carefully; seeking out a birth attendant with a low cesarean rate; using a labor partner; and forgoing all unnecessary interventions in a normal labor.

If you've chosen your birth attendant carefully, you should trust that you will not have a cesarean unless it is absolutely necessary. As one mother said, "We knew a cesarean had to be done because we'd tried everything else. I have no regrets or afterthoughts."

When a cesarean does need to be performed, it's rarely such an emergency that you have no choices at all. An excellent pamphlet available from Pennypress (see Resources) discusses many of the options you should think about in advance of a cesarean.

Two choices you should be able to discuss if your cesarean is not a dire emergency are the types of incision and anesthesia you receive. A bikini cut, done just under the top of your pubic-hair line, is almost always possible unless your cesarean needs to be done very quickly, or your baby's or placenta's position makes it unsafe. This type of incision will reduce your blood loss and discomfort while also minimizing your chances of getting a postpartum infection. It's also much less disfiguring than the vertical or "classical" incision.

For future deliveries, though, it's the uterine cut that really matters. Today almost all cesareans are performed with a horizontal low-cervical incision that is perfectly reliable and needn't be considered a weak spot in future vaginal births.

As far as anesthesia is concerned, a regional block such as a spinal or epidural (see chapter 18), which will numb you from the breast down, is a better choice than general anesthesia, which is usually reserved for the most acute emergency situations and which poses more risks for both you and your baby.

18
Medical Aids

Your obstetrician believes her patients should try to give birth with as little medical intervention as possible, while your friend's doctor reassures his patients "not to worry," because he will make sure they're "comfortable" during labor. Your sister's nurse-midwife says that hardly any of her patients need painkillers. But a local group of doctors requires their patients to come to a mandatory lecture by an anesthesiologist who touts the epidural block as the "Cadillac of obstetric anesthesia." With such basic disagreements among professionals, how can you choose which medication, if any, you should have during labor?

The first thing to realize is that you *do* have a choice, even if your choice is to leave all decision-making up to your doctor or midwife. Of course, you should trust your birth practitioner's judgment so that you can rely on that person's decisions in a medical emergency. But most decisions about medication during childbirth do not need to be made on an emergency basis. The nonemergency decisions are really yours to make.

Since any medication taken during your labor has the potential to affect your body, your baby, your labor, and your experience of the birth, you owe it to yourself and to your baby to learn as much as you can about the pros and cons of medication. Then your choices will be well-informed.

Medication: Weighing the Risks

Many women who spend their pregnancies being suitably cautious about taking medication somehow assume they have entered a "free zone" when they come to the hospital in labor. You shouldn't—your fetus *in utero* is affected by any medications you take.

A baby who receives your medications during labor and delivery but is born before he passes them back to you through the placenta inherits the task of breaking down and excreting the drugs himself. While you can do this relatively easily, your newborn baby's immature liver and kidneys may have a harder time doing the job. Your baby could be born with no apparent effects from the medication. Or he could display problems at birth ranging from the subtle—fussiness, diminished muscle tone, or a temporary lack of interest in sounds or sights—to the more serious—such as respiratory depression.

The American Academy of Pediatrics Committee on Drugs states that there is no drug which, when taken by or administered to a childbearing woman, has been proven safe for her unborn child. Not proven safe doesn't mean the same thing as proven unsafe. It simply means that no one, no matter how well-intentioned, can guarantee that your baby will experience no ill effects from the medications you take during labor.

Many labor medications, for example, can cause hypotension, a drop in your blood pressure. When your blood pressure falls, blood is diverted from the uterus, a "nonessential" organ, and your baby may be temporarily deprived of a healthy oxygen supply. Medications may alter your ability to concentrate and work alertly with your contractions, or they may impair your ability to push your baby out without the aid of forceps. Sometimes a "simple" medication can be the first step to a whole host of obstetrical interventions and procedures which make the birth very different from the experience you had anticipated. Getting an epidural, for example, means you must labor in bed. Other birth medications may cause nausea or leave you with a bad headache.

Many people assume that the more pain relief a woman gets, the more positive her birth experience will be. But this isn't necessarily true. The way a woman gives birth profoundly affects her self-image. A mother who can experience her labor with minimal or no medication usually forgets the pain quickly and may feel afterward as though she mastered a difficult challenge. A large-scale *Parents* magazine poll found that, compared to women who took no medication during vaginal deliveries, medicated women were significantly more likely to feel they would want to do things differently next time.

Medication: Weighing the Benefits

Women's goals for their birth experiences differ, and so do their pain thresholds and their labors. Despite the best intentions, births don't always happen as planned. Although you should be encouraged to experience birth without medication if this is desirable *and* possible for you, some labors are actually helped by medication.

As you may recall from chapter 1, intense pain and anxiety can stimulate catecholamines like adrenaline in the mother's circulation. Catecholamines cause dysfunctional labor, reducing uterine blood flow and thereby decreasing your baby's oxygen supply. If you cannot relax by nonchemical means, medication may benefit you and your baby because relaxation enhances uterine circulation. Medication may also offer you a much-needed respite if your labor is temporarily unproductive or if it is excruciatingly painful over a long period. Getting some relief can allow you to regain the energy you'll need to push your baby out. If you have a cesarean delivery or a delivery requiring forceps, anesthesia will be used.

Medication for Labor

Medications used during labor and birth fall into two major categories: *analgesics,* which offer partial relief to the conscious patient by increasing her pain threshold, and which include narcotics and low-dose inhalation agents; and *anesthetics,* which offer a woman complete pain relief or unconsciousness by blocking nerve impulses to her brain. Sedatives (barbiturates) and tranquilizers give no relief from pain, but may be employed in the first stage of labor to promote relaxation, combat anxiety, induce sleep, or boost the action of analgesic medications.

During the first stage of labor, your uterus contracts at gradually decreasing intervals, but with increasing strength and length, until the cervix or neck portion of your uterus is completely dilated and you can begin to push your baby out into the world. This stage lasts an average of 12 to 18 hours for a first baby (less for subsequent births), but it can be much longer or shorter. It is a time when some women may need medication to cope with the increasingly powerful sensations of stretching, pressure, and, possibly, back pain.

Very Early Labor.   You'll usually spend this period at home, relaxing in a familiar environment. However, sometimes a woman is hospitalized in early labor, or even before her contractions have begun, perhaps because her membranes have ruptured prematurely.

If you have a lengthy but unproductive early labor and are utterly exhausted from missing a night or more of sleep, you may get sleeping medication, orally or in an injection, to help you regain some energy before heavy labor begins. Such relief can also encourage your labor to become more effective.

Sedatives (barbiturates), such as Nembutal or Seconal, may be used alone or in combination with a narcotic such as morphine. One mother who was given Seconal with morphine says, "It was just what I needed after missing two nights of sleep. After a few hours of dozing between contractions, my labor perked up and I was able to have a spontaneous delivery."

Because barbiturates are not easily excreted by you or your baby, both of you may be somewhat depressed as an aftereffect of such medication. Unlike a narcotic-induced depression, which can be reversed by Narcan (a narcotic antagonist), barbiturate-induced depression must wear off on its own. You might find yourself sleepy and unable to cope with contractions when labor does begin, and you may have a "hangover" the next day. Your baby could show delayed sucking and altered behavioral responses until he is able to metabolize and excrete the medication.

Midlabor.   For difficulty in coping with strong contractions during the middle of labor, you may be offered narcotics, tranquilizers, anesthetics such as a paracervical or epidural block, or—much less frequently—inhalation analgesia. Variations exist, so be sure and find out just what is offered at your own hospital.

Demerol (meperidine) is the *narcotic* most commonly used during labor. Given in an injection—usually in the hip—it takes 40 to 50 minutes to take full effect, and the pain relief lasts for three to four hours. If the dose is given intravenously, you will feel the effects within five to ten minutes, and they should last for about one hour. Often part of the dose is given in the shot and part into your IV to combine the quick onset of the intravenous infusion with the longer-acting effects of the intramuscular injection.

In some hospitals, substitute narcotics may be used in place of Demerol:

- Dilaudid (hydromorophone)
- Sublimaze (fentanyl)
- Stadol (butorphanol)
- Nubain (nalbuphine)
- Talwin (pentazocine)

Ask your own caregiver which narcotic is typically used for labor in your hospital, and be sure to inquire about its length of action, effectiveness, and side effects.

Years ago, women in labor routinely got large doses of narcotics, and maternal side effects such as lowered blood pressure, nausea, vomiting, dizziness, dry mouth, and respiratory depression were much more common. Today's dosages are smaller and these side effects occur less frequently.

In doses small enough to be considered safe for laboring women, narcotics do not afford total pain relief. But they can often "take the edge off" contractions, allowing you to relax more readily during and especially between the contractions. As one mother puts it, "The shot made me high and didn't really take the pain away, but it enabled me to 'distance' myself from it."

Narcotics, especially Demerol, may be mixed with a *tranquilizer* such as Vistaril, Phenergan, or Largon, in order to prevent maternal nausea and decrease the amount of Demerol given. Tranquilizers cross the placenta rapidly, but specific fetal effects are hard to isolate because tranquilizers rarely get administered except in combination with narcotics that have side effects of their own.

You probably won't get narcotics before around four centimeters of dilatation, because these painkillers can slow down your labor. The most serious fetal side effect, depressed respiration, depends on many factors: the timing of administration, the amount of the drug or its metabolites left in the fetal circulation at birth, the baby's gestational age (because premies are more subject to respiratory depression, their mothers are seldom offered narcotics in labor), the baby's weight, and the length and difficulty of your labor.

In a few hospitals you may be offered the opportunity to give yourself narcotic medication whenever you need it, in limited, preset doses, through an infusion pump on an intravenous line. One research study showed that women getting the narcotic Nubain this way used one-third less medication than women requesting medication in shots and reported greater satisfaction and significantly less nausea and drowsiness.

Since the projected timing of the birth must remain an educated guess, at times a baby emerges with too much narcotic in his system. In these cases, the baby may get a shot of Narcan, a narcotic antagonist, as soon as he is born. Narcan can immediately reverse the neonatal respiratory depression caused by narcotics given to a mother too close to birth.

Women vary in their reactions to narcotics. A woman who expects total pain relief will probably be disappointed. And some women don't appreciate the "fuzzy" feeling narcotics can give: "It made everything seem unfocused and unclear," says one mother, "and it didn't lessen my pain. I still felt scared and panicky, but light-headed, as though I'd had several glasses of wine." Another woman appreciated the injection she received during a lengthy labor, saying, "It was just what I needed to give me the strength to keep going. After the shot I could rest and get on top of the breathing. It allowed me to gear up for the pushing stage."

Inhalation agents, such as nitrous oxide and Penthrane, are infrequently used in labor in the United States, though they are common in Great Britain. With proper administration these agents do not lead to respiratory depression and they usually have no negative effect on labor. Anesthetics administered in a subanesthetic dose, nitrous oxide and Penthrane offer stronger analgesia than the more commonly used narcotics at current doses.

Inhalation agents are usually self-administered by the woman, who breathes in a concentration of gas and oxygen from a hand-held mask. When you begin to feel light-headed, you drop the mask and immediately revive.

The major drawback to this form of pain relief is inadvertent overdose, which can lead to vomiting and aspiration. Penthrane may also cause renal damage in an excessive dosage. Of course, inhalation agents should be used only at hospitals where trained assistants and appropriate apparatus are available.

Two regional anesthetics may be used to alleviate pain during labor: the paracervical block and the epidural block. The paracervical block can be given by your doctor or by a house physician in the labor room. This shot is injected with a very long needle into areas corresponding with four o'clock and eight o'clock on the cervix. The tip of the needle injects a local anesthetic into the rim of the cervix. Complete pain relief for dilatation lasts about 45 to 90 minutes and the shot can be repeated from about four centimeters to about eight centimeters dilatation.

In recent years, however, the paracervical block has fallen out of favor because it frequently slows down the fetal heart rate. At most hospitals, in fact, the paracervical block has completely disappeared in favor of the epidural block.

The epidural has been designated the Cadillac of obstetric anesthesia because, compared to narcotics and inhalation analgesia, it offers almost complete pain relief during labor. Sometimes a mother will find an epidural invaluable for reducing involuntary pushing against an incompletely dilated cervix. And an extremely anxious patient making no progress in labor may advance very rapidly after she gets an epidural. Indeed, epidurals are so effective at relieving labor pain that they are used at some hospitals for more than three-quarters of all deliveries.

Because the epidural requires special skills to administer and monitor, it is not available at all hospitals. To avoid its potential side effects, the epidural must be given by a trained anesthesiologist or nurse-anesthetist who will monitor you carefully afterwards.

Unlike the spinal, which goes through the membrane encasing the spinal fluid and is used only for delivery, the epidural is injected outside the dura, or spinal membrane. It can be readministered throughout labor through a small, soft catheter left in place by the anesthesiologist. At many hospitals nowadays, epidurals are given by means of a continuous infusion, rather than a dose that needs to be repeated. The dose and concentration of medication can be varied to produce any level of analgesia from minimal to profound.

Before an epidural is administered, you will be given an IV to insure that any blood pressure drop caused by dilatation of your blood vessels can be rapidly alleviated by the administration of fluids or medication. Your lower back will be cleaned with a disinfectant and a needle will be injected about two inches into the epidural space surrounding your spinal membrane, an area rich in nerve endings. A small, flexible catheter is then threaded through the needle, left in your back, and covered by a sterile dressing. The needle is then removed. The catheter tube will be brought up over your shoulder and taped to your chest, allowing the medication to be continually infused or repeated as needed.

The initial dose takes five to ten minutes to take effect (the effect peaks at twenty minutes) and lasts from 45 minutes to two hours. Women getting a continuous infusion may continue to receive medication through the catheter until the birth.

The vast majority of women obtain excellent pain relief with the epidural. A few women, however, fail to get any relief from it. Others experience a "window" or gap in the anesthetized area, and for about three percent the epidural "takes" on one side only.

Recently anesthesiologists have begun to mix small doses of narcotics with the dilute anesthetic solution in continuous epidural infusions. Dr. Richard E. Gelfand, head of obstetric anesthesia at Evanston Hospital, says, "We get raves on these new epidurals. The patients are not nearly as numb. They get serious pain relief from the narcotics, but now they can move more easily in bed and push much more effectively because they still feel the sensations of pressure."

Research from Great Britain suggests that mothers do indeed prefer epidurals when narcotics are added to the anesthetic. Women whose epidurals included narcotics reported greater self-control, less leg weakness and shivering, and less unpleasant numbness than did women who got epidurals containing only anesthetic. Perhaps more important, the group with narcotics in their epidurals experienced half the rate of forceps deliveries and one-sixth the rate of rotational midforceps deliveries that the standard epidural group experienced.

The addition of narcotics into epidurals does appear to afford good pain relief while preserving a mother's ability to move in bed and push effectively. Thus far, clinical experience with epidural narcotics is positive. Dr. Gelfand says, "The narcotic never or almost never depresses the baby or mother."

But this technique is relatively new and it is not completely free of side effects. Epidural narcotics frequently lead to maternal itching or urinary retention. In addition, narcotics administered in the epidural space could cause respiratory depression in the baby or the mother. After a delivery with epidural narcotics, a mother should be observed carefully for 24 hours to make sure she does not get a delayed onset of respiratory depression.

Opinions on epidurals differ. A labor with no or very little sensation may be one woman's ideal but another woman's disappointment. For one second-time mother, the epidural "worked like a charm. I felt pressure but no pain from the contractions. I talked freely and laughed with my husband, comparing it to my previous 'natural' childbirth. Compared to that, this was a pain-free birth with no bad memories, no sweating, no exhaustion during and afterwards."

An epidural carries many potential medical side effects, but these can be prevented or treated. Your blood pressure may drop, for example, threatening your baby's well-being. Any woman who gets an epidural, however, will already be receiving IV fluids to guard against this possibility and to treat it if it occurs. Your blood pressure will be monitored quite frequently during a labor under epidural block—every minute or two for the first ten minutes and then every five to ten minutes until the block wears off—and you will usually be encouraged to lie on your side. You will have to stay in bed, but will be encouraged to turn from side to side to avoid a one-sided block.

An epidural may also slow down your labor. If this happens, Pitocin can be given through your IV to stimulate labor. Naturally, a fetal monitor must be used to check your baby's heart rate and the contractions you may no longer feel. Difficulty in urinating, more frequent after regional anesthesia, can be dealt with by catheterization. If you get a urinary infection, it can be treated with antibiotics. If your temperature rises—more common under an epidural—you can get sponged or fanned to cool off.

An epidural can be administered at around three or four centimeters of dilatation with women who have had babies before, but should not be given before five or six centimeters to women having their first babies. Given too early, the epidural is more likely to slow down labor.

Indeed, a retrospective study published in the *American Journal of Obstetrics and Gynecology* in 1989 revealed that nearly three times as many first-time mothers with slow labors who took epidurals had cesareans for failure to progress as did women with slow labors who did not take epidurals. Discussing his research, Dr. James A. Thorp of St. Luke's Hospital in Kansas City, Missouri, said, "There are many mechanisms by which epidural analgesia could increase the frequency of cesarean section for dystocia [failure to progress in labor]. All the following potential mechanisms have a basis in the literature: decreased uterine activity, prolongation of the first stage of labor, relaxation of the pelvic diaphragm predisposing to minor malpresentation, decreased maternal urge to push, decreased maternal ability to push, prolonged second stage of labor, and increased risk of instrumental vaginal delivery, a procedure that is unlikely to be performed for medicolegal reasons."

Long-term side effects of epidurals are unknown. But a British study recently suggested that epidurals during labor may predispose new mothers to getting backaches. When a large number of mothers were sent questionnaires 12 months to nine years after giving birth, 18.9 percent of mothers who'd had epidurals reported backaches that began within three months of delivery and lasted more than six weeks, compared to only 10 percent of women who had not gotten epidurals. The researchers theorized that the muscle relaxation of pregnancy and the abolition of pain during labor may have combined to allow mothers with epidurals to lie for long periods of time in potentially damaging positions.

The epidural, which effectively relieves pain, also renders the birth a high-technology affair, managed by the medical staff with the aid of much modern machinery. A new mother recalls, "I had no sense of achievement. The labor was taken away from me, and the birth—

well, it was like watching someone give birth on TV."

If you have an epidural for labor, you can still participate in the birth, but more or less actively depending on the type of epidural you have had and whether it has worn off. Traditional anesthetic epidurals are usually allowed to wear off for pushing, while epidurals with narcotics may be kept running until the baby is born.

Because the anesthetic is transferred through the placenta, your baby may experience some temporary side effects. Irritability, poor sucking, and diminished muscle tone have been reported in some babies whose mothers were given an epidural block. These side effects, however, were associated with an anesthetic agent no longer in current use for continuous epidurals.

Infrequently—about once or twice in a hundred epidurals—the needle for the epidural inadvertently punctures the membrane encasing the spinal fluid. Usually a test dose will disclose if the needle is in the wrong place. But if the drug is injected, you will temporarily be paralyzed, a frightening event. A woman who has received this so-called wet epidural is likely to get a "spinal headache," a usually painful but temporary and treatable aftereffect (see page 219). Once in a while the medication rises in the epidural space, interfering with a woman's ability to breathe and necessitating temporary mechanical assistance. Quite infrequently, convulsions occur as a result of too high a level of anesthesia. As with any local anesthetic, it is possible to have a serious toxic reaction if too much medication is given or if medication is injected into a blood vessel; this, too, is very rare.

Medication for Birth

Pushing lasts an average of about 80 minutes for a first baby; it is shorter for subsequent babies. Medication for delivery ranges from general anesthesia, which renders a woman unconscious, to no anesthetic at all. The analgesics, tranquilizers, and sedatives that may be used during the first stage of labor are not offered close to the birth. Sometimes, because of extreme anxiety or a desire to be dissociated from the birth, a woman will prefer to be completely numbed for her baby's delivery. Women whose mothers were routinely "knocked out" even for vaginal deliveries frequently assume that the baby's birth must be the most painful part. It's not. Women who have felt the extraordinary sensations of giving birth report that the baby's birth is a joyous climax to labor.

Vaginal Delivery.   The intense stretching sensations of pushing are unusual—"preposterous" more than painful, says Sheila Kitzinger—but it is powerful and exciting to be involved in such a great effort. To the extent that you can participate in the birth of your baby, you'll enjoy the rewards of your active involvement.

For the majority of women who deliver vaginally, pain relief during birth will be needed only for the repair of the episiotomy, performed right before the baby emerges. If an episiotomy is to be done or if you experience some lacerations at birth that require suturing afterward, a pudendal block to numb your vagina or an injection of local anesthetic may be given into your perineum. A local can be injected right before the birth, or even afterward, because the distension caused by the baby's head will numb your perineum for the minute or two before birth. If you are trying to deliver without an episiotomy, nurse-midwife Nancy Fleming suggests that you *not* get a shot of local anesthetic before delivery. Women in her study on episiotomy were significantly more likely to tear if they got a shot before delivery.

No specific fetal effects have been documented from the pudendal block or from the local. But critics warn that these blocks—usually considered innocuous—should be employed cautiously before birth, because large amounts of local anesthetic are used and the medication crosses the placenta quickly.

A pudendal block is given in two steps with a long needle through the vagina. The tip of the needle injects a local anesthetic into the pudendal nerve, first on one side and then the other. A pudendal block numbs your perineum and the lower portion of your vagina. Unlike the caudal or epidural, the pudendal may be administered by your own doctor. It should not numb your legs, though some women experience the temporary numbing of a leg as a side effect.

If you get a pudendal block, you may feel the baby in the birth canal, but you will not have all the sensations of his movement down and out. You may lose your bearing-down reflex, but you should be able to push well from memory. If you need a low- or outlet-forceps delivery, the pudendal may afford you sufficient anesthesia.

Local perineal infiltration offers the least amount of interference with the natural process of birth and your active participation in it. Your doctor may inject a local anesthetic into one or more spots in the perineum near the entrance to the vagina, either before the episiotomy or immediately after the birth. One experienced mother reports, "The local was less painful in administration and more effective than the pudendal I had for my first birth. I was happy to play such an active part in this birth. It was exhilarating to feel my baby moving down the birth canal, and words can't describe the wonder of her birth."

Preexisting medical conditions such as heart disease may prevent you from participating in active pushing. And some women who are able to push find it to be excruciatingly painful or frustratingly non-productive, because of the size of their baby or their baby's position in the birth canal. Some babies, for example, need a midforceps rotation in order to emerge. For a woman who needs or wants to be numbed and assisted with her delivery, a saddle, epidural, or caudal block may be given.

Spinals are rarely used for vaginal deliveries now that epidurals and caudals are so common. However, at some hospitals, a type of spinal called a saddle block—numbing only the parts of your body that would touch a saddle—may be given for a difficult delivery if very rapid anesthesia is necessary or if an epidural or caudal presents problems in administration. Since effective bearing down is impossible after a spinal block, a spinal should be given only when the baby's head is visible at the vaginal opening.

Like the saddle block, epidurals and caudals are usually given and monitored by an anesthesiologist because of potential problems such as a decrease in the mother's blood pressure. Which type of block you are offered depends on the training of the staff where you are having your baby. Epidurals and caudals have a similar effect—the numbing of your body from the waist down—though the caudal is administered at the base of the spine and the epidural is administered at waist level. In most hospitals, the epidural has replaced the caudal because it is more reliable, easier to administer, and uses less medication. The intent with either block is to numb the pelvic area, but numbness usually spreads to the legs and abdominal muscles as well.

For a caudal or epidural, you may need to be separated from your labor partner for the administration, though this is not the case in every hospital. Since it takes some time for the medication to become effective, your support person may have a waiting period before you can be reunited for the delivery.

Once the medication takes effect, your urge to push will probably disappear. Some women find this numbness disconcerting: "I didn't know when I was having a contraction and I couldn't feel myself pushing," complained one woman who disliked the loss of sensation.

But you can push from memory, the same way you can chew gum even after getting Novocain at the dentist's office. Try looking in the mirror to see the effects of your pushing. Some women do this quite well and report a lot of satisfaction at knowing their efforts helped to get their baby born. You may be profoundly grateful for the numbing effects of the epidural block, as was this mother:

I'd pushed for three hours, but the baby hadn't come down very far at all. I wouldn't have requested an epidural simply to have a painless delivery, but it was obvious I wasn't going to deliver in a reasonable time by continuing to push. With the epidural, I was numb from mid-abdomen down, but I remembered how to push and I still could push on signal while the doctor pulled gently with forceps. Psychologically, it was great. I knew birth was coming soon. I was not in pain, and I could enjoy the birth.

Because both the caudal and the epidural provide complete relaxation of the pelvic floor muscles, a baby may fail to rotate into the proper position for birth. Some babies will need to have the assistance of a midforceps rotation to be born. Other babies—about half of those whose mothers have a caudal or epidural—will need low or outlet forceps just to ease their heads out once they have reached the perineum. The use of forceps requires a larger episiotomy, which may increase the mother's postpartum pain (see chapter 20).

After the Birth.   While narcotics, sedatives, or tranquilizers may be offered after the delivery, they can make you feel groggy and uninterested in your baby, who is usually most alert and responsive for the first one or two hours after birth. Breathing and relaxation techniques can help, and mild painkillers may be used if necessary. A warm blanket alleviates the chills and shakes so many women get after delivery.

Cesarean Delivery.   When your baby must be born by cesarean, you will obviously need more extensive anesthesia than for a vaginal birth. Though some hospitals use general anesthesia for a majority of surgical births, in many hospitals generals are reserved for those situations when the speed of anesthetic effect outweighs the disadvantages of the mother's being asleep for the birth. A general anesthetic may also be preferable if back problems or other maternal conditions render the use of regional anesthesia impossible or unsafe, or if you prefer not to be awake for the delivery.

The main disadvantage of general anesthesia is the rare but quite serious risk of a mother's aspirating vomit because her gag reflex has been put to sleep. Furthermore, babies born under general anesthesia are more likely to be depressed, particularly if the delivery is not performed as soon as possible—usually within five to ten minutes—after the administration of the medication. Because some general anesthetics interfere with uterine contractions, postpartum blood loss may be greater. If the mother sleeps through the delivery with a general, she will be groggy for the important postpartum hours. Her partner is usually not permitted to be present for the birth, though in some hospitals, if general anesthesia is given for a nonemergency case, her partner is invited to be there as the mother's "eyes and ears" when the baby is born. When a general anesthetic wears off, the onset of pain can be sudden and overwhelming. New mothers seem to take a bit longer to recover from cesareans performed under a general anesthetic.

An anesthesiologist will administer general anesthesia in several steps. Remember that your baby will be born within the first few minutes after the anesthetic takes effect. First, oxygen will be given by mask to boost your baby's oxygen supply. The mask may have a plastic smell, but it is not the anesthetic, so take good, deep whiffs. You will usually go to sleep shortly after Pentothal and/or another barbiturate is administered through your IV; you'll also be given succinylcholine, a muscle relaxant. At this point, firm but gentle pressure will be applied over your neck by an assistant to help prevent the possibility of your choking.

As soon as you are unconscious, a long plastic tube will most likely be placed down your throat and into your trachea to administer the anesthetic gas, usually nitrous oxide. The endotracheal tube is usually used in place of a mask because it prevents the danger of your inhaling food or gastric acid while you are asleep. Your baby will usually be delivered within two to ten minutes, and the suturing will take 30 or more minutes afterward.

During the surgery, you will remain unconscious and will not feel anything. In the recovery room, you will slowly come back to consciousness. You may be groggy and sleepy for about a day after the birth. Most women completely excrete the anesthetic within 24 hours.

If you do not need a general anesthetic, either a spinal or an epidural may be used. Both afford sufficient anesthesia so that you will not feel pain during the surgery. These blocks involve placement of a needle in the mother's back and the injection of a local anesthetic. To get a spinal or an epidural, the mother lies on her side with her knees drawn up, or sits up and leans over, in order to provide maximum separation between the vertebrae in her spine.

Because the epidural is a little more difficult to administer, at some hospitals only the spinal will be available. The spinal is also preferable to the epidural when speed is essential, because it takes effect several minutes faster than an epidural. For example, when fetal distress has occurred but the baby is not in immediate jeopardy, the spinal may be a better choice.

Some doctors prefer the spinal for other reasons. It is easier to give and more reliably effective than the epidural, and it gives more intense anesthesia with a much smaller dose of medication. There is less transfer of the medication across the placenta, and there is a smaller risk of the mother's incurring a toxic reaction to the anesthetic.

The spinal does have some drawbacks, however. "Spinal headaches," thought to be caused by the leakage of spinal fluid at the puncture site, are less common now that smaller-gauge needles are used, but about five to ten in a hundred women receiving spinals still get headaches, even with the tiniest needles.

Contrary to popular belief, bed rest after a spinal does not reduce the incidence of spinal headaches, so getting up and walking after the delivery is usually allowed once the block wears off. But if you do get a headache, you will probably be advised to remain in bed and may be treated with fluids, analgesics, and an abdominal binder, to decrease the leakage of spinal fluid. If these measures fail to relieve your headache, it can be treated by an "epidural blood patch," so-called because a small amount of your blood is injected into the epidural space at the site of the spinal; this usually provides immediate relief by clotting to seal the hole.

An epidural may be chosen for several reasons. Maternal hypotension (lowered blood pressure) comes on more gradually with an epidural than with a spinal, making the drop in blood pressure easier to treat and leading less frequently to maternal nausea and vomiting. If the spinal wears off during surgery or fails to take effect, a general must be given, whereas an epidural can be "topped up" because the catheter remains in place. With an epidural, a woman's legs are merely numbed, not always paralyzed, and mothers experience less difficulty breathing during the surgery. Women who have cesareans under an epidural report feeling some of the tugging sensations of the baby's birth. This is not painful and it provides some women with more of a sense that they have been involved in the birth process. Finally, if the epidural is administered without problems, a woman is not at risk for a headache after the birth. If an epidural is inadvertently injected into the dura, recent research indicates that injecting a saline solution through the epidural catheter after the anesthetic wears off can significantly reduce the incidence of spinal headaches.

A newly delivered mother tells how the anesthesiologist administered the epidural for her cesarean:

> After twelve hours of labor, my cervix would dilate no more than eight centimeters and the baby's heart rate indicated some fetal distress; a cesarean section was decided upon. It was hard to sit upright for the epidural because I had a contraction and the urge to push while he was working on me, and it was vital that I remain motionless. But when he

finally finished, I felt better almost immediately. It was heaven going from exhausting, nonproductive contractions to warm, tingling relief.

Rarely, a doctor prefers merely to inject the woman's abdomen with a local anesthetic in order to minimize the mother's and the baby's exposure to anesthesia. Again, be sure to find out what's available and recommended at your hospital. It's usually a good idea to get the type of anesthesia your hospital's staff is most competent and experienced at giving.

Use Medication Only If You Need It, but Don't Feel Guilty If You Do. During pregnancy, share your goals for the birth with your doctor or midwife. Your medical caregivers as well as your labor companion are important partners in helping you achieve your goals for the birth. If you prefer not to use medication, you should be able to express this without being made to feel that you are setting yourself up for martyrdom on the one hand or failure on the other. You should let your birth attendant know if there are any particular medications you want or do not want to use during labor. Frank discussion can help to create an atmosphere of mutual trust and understanding should the need for medication arise during labor.

When you get to the hospital, you may want to ask or remind your doctor and nurses not to offer you medication for pain relief. This puts the burden on you to ask only for medications you feel you need, and it also takes away the burden of saying no at a time when you'll probably be feeling very vulnerable.

Don't feel guilty if you decide to ask for medication, but it's best not to take it at the very first sign of discomfort. If you wait until you really need the assistance, you'll have the feeling that you've given your all to the experience. At times, a lengthy plateau during labor may be helped by the administration of medication. But if you ask for medication right away, you'll never know how you would have done without it. Don't ever make decisions about medication during a contraction; do so in the rest period between contractions.

Remember, too, to be examined just before taking any medication during labor. Sometimes just being told of your progress provides enough of a boost to make taking medication seem superfluous. Often, a woman who asks for medication is really asking for reassurance from her labor supporters that she is "doing all right." Given with sympathy and confidence, such reassurance can provide as much pain relief as most injections.

Much has been said about the guilt a woman will feel if she plans for birth without medication and eventually needs to have it. But when you consider thoroughly beforehand the benefits as well as the risks of medication, you can understand that in certain situations (different, perhaps, for each woman) childbirth medication may be necessary or desirable. Using this information should give you the feeling that you are working with your caregivers in order to make the best possible decisions for your baby, your labor, and yourself.

19

Is Birth Painful for the Baby, Too?

If you find your labor contractions painful, what must they feel like to your baby? Despite the impossibility of interviewing a newborn, plenty of imaginative speculation exists about what babies feel during birth.

In 1920, Joseph B. DeLee wrote in the *American Journal of Obstetrics and Gynecology* that labor felt to the baby like having his head crushed in a door. From the mother's perspective, DeLee compared giving birth to falling on a pitchfork! Because he thought the birth process was so dangerous for both mother and baby, DeLee advocated sedation, ether, forceps, episiotomy, and manual removal of the placenta after birth. Although DeLee's article had a major influence on obstetrical practice for decades after it was published, many of the very interventions he advocated are now believed to *increase* trauma to mothers and babies.

Half a century later, Frederick Leboyer's *Birth Without Violence* purported to describe birth from the baby's point of view. Leboyer's imagery is even more shocking than DeLee's. Birth, according to Leboyer, is "the torture of an innocent." Leboyer calls the laboring mother "a monster" and "the enemy." The newborn infant is said to be "crazed with pain."

Who wouldn't be crazed with pain in the situation Leboyer describes? "The monster," he writes, "drives the baby lower still. And not satisfied with crushing it, [she] twists it in a refinement of cruelty. . . . Hell is what the infant must suffer through to arrive here among us. Its flames assail the child from every direction; they burn the eyes, the skin, penetrate down through the flesh; they devour. This fire is what the baby feels as the air rushes into the lungs."

Well, maybe. . . . But then again, probably not. For normal vaginal birth to have evolved as "torture" for the baby seems highly unlikely. Actually, observers of birth usually remark on how untraumatized and alert most babies appear immediately afterwards.

Stress hormones normally rise to very high levels in newborn babies. Described in chapter 1, these hormones—catecholamines—usually prepare a person to fight or flee from a threat. In an adult, high concentrations typically indicate severe distress. But the particular hormone the infant produces (noradrenaline) *reduces* his heart rate, thereby protecting him from oxygen deprivation during labor. That's probably why so many babies who show heart rate decelerations during labor are born in excellent condition.

The surge of catecholamines that protects your infant from oxygen deprivation during labor also initiates several changes which prepare his lungs to function more adequately after birth. Babies who are delivered by cesarean section without experiencing labor miss this catecholamine surge and consequently suffer more often from breathing problems at birth. Far from being a stress to your baby, the catecholamines he produces during labor actually *promote* his adaptation to the outside world.

Catecholamines also enhance your baby's appearance and alertness after birth. Because of these hormones, your baby's pupils dilate. This gives him that wide-awake look most new parents find irresistible.

Birth, then, is probably much less traumatic for your baby than you may have feared. Babies are, however, highly sensitive to pain at birth. Fanciful though it was, Leboyer's book encouraged the gentle treatment of newborns at a time when their ability to feel at all was totally disregarded.

Easing Birth for Your Baby

Because your baby can see, hear, and feel at birth, the kind of obstetric care that meets your own needs will usually lead to sensitive care for your new baby, too. For example, very bright lights which would be irritating to anybody's eyes should certainly be turned down as long as your perineum is well illuminated.

Actually, unborn babies are not really floating in the dark. In late pregnancy, they can see a sort of rosy glow through the thinned uterus and stretched skin of the abdomen. Fetuses have been shown to respond to bright lights as well as to loud sounds. Once your baby is born, shade his eyes from the delivery room light if it's too bright for him to open them. If he keeps his eyes closed, try holding him a little more upright. Like a doll baby, your newborn's eyes will close when he's lying down and open when he's brought to a more vertical position.

You don't need to worry about being silent at birth, as Dr. Leboyer has advocated. Your spontaneous greetings won't hurt your baby's ears and you probably couldn't stop yourself from making noise even if you tried. At the moment of my son's birth, I wondered who was squealing with delight until I realized I was the noisy one! My husband was cheering too.

Contrary to what you might imagine, your unborn baby hardly awaits his debut in a quiet environment. According to a book called *The Amazing Newborn*, researchers who placed tiny microphones along a six- to seven-month-old fetus detected maternal noises at a volume slightly less than that of a busy city street! Novelist Robertson Davies has written, "We're carried in the womb in a positive hub-bub—the tom-tom of the heart, the croaking and gurgling of the guts, which must sound like the noise of the rigging on a sailing ship, and a mother's loud laughter. . . . Silence is entirely an acquired taste." Because your baby has been exposed to the loud sounds of your body's workings for all these months, and to the sound of your voice, he's quite prepared to hear your spontaneous greetings.

If your baby is delivered onto your abdomen or thigh, and you're in a semi-upright position, you'll be well situated to greet him with your fingertips. You don't need to be taught how to touch him, nor is touch a strange, new sensation for your baby. He's been surrounded for months by the continuous touch of the amniotic fluid and he's just had a great massage. He's primed for your touch.

After your baby's first cry, which forces his lungs open, he's apt to quiet and look around, quite peaceful and content in his new world. For most new babies, the first hour after birth is a wonderful period of alertness. If you hold him with his face about eight to twelve inches from yours, your baby will focus on your eyes and will turn toward the sound of your voice. He already knows your voice, and, perhaps because of this, responds more readily to high-pitched voices. Fathers may quite naturally find themselves talking to their new babies in a falsetto range.

If the delivery room is cool—and it usually is kept somewhat cool for the comfort of the gowned and gloved attendants—your baby may lose body heat rapidly. Several studies have shown, however, that if you and your baby are warmed by a blanket or a portable heater, your naked baby will stay just as warm against your body as he would if he were removed to a heated crib. So if you'd like your baby in your arms immediately after birth and he's in good condition, there's no real need for him to be anyplace else. In many hospitals, newborns are given a tiny knit cap to minimize heat loss from their heads.

The idea of bathing the baby shortly after birth has been hotly debated. Many doctors express a concern that the baby might become chilled. Because a newborn baby has a large area of exposed skin relative to his body mass, he does lose heat more rapidly than a larger person; what's more, he can't yet shiver to conserve heat. But, if the room can be warmed and if an insulated tub is available, your baby may enjoy his first bath in the delivery room.

Mothers who can see and touch their new baby in this first bath often say it enhances the magical feelings of the birth:

> The lights were dimmed in the delivery room and immediately after the baby was born she was placed on my belly. Chad and I cleaned her off. Dr. Stein offered Chad the scissors to cut the cord, which he did. Then the nurse drew a warm bath for Chad to bathe Karen. I held her hand in the bath. It was fascinating how calm she became in the bath. She stopped crying and just stared at her father.

Some newborn babies, however, don't like a bath, as one new mother discovered to her chagrin:

> She was very alert at birth and able to lift her head and look around. She seemed quite calm and interested in what was going on. My husband cut the umbilical cord under the doctor's direction. The bath was prepared and when my husband took the baby and gently placed her in the warm water, she gave a loud wail of displeasure. So much for Leboyer!

If your baby is perfectly content lying against your abdomen and looking around, beginning perhaps to nuzzle at your nipple, it may be superfluous to plop him into a tub of water. After all, he's already made the necessary transition to our environment of air. But, if the bath sounds appealing to you and your doctors and nurses are enthusiastic, you and your baby may find it a very pleasurable event.

In most hospitals, it's standard practice to forgo tub baths for newborns for several days, until their umbilical cords have fallen off. Instead, they're usually sponged off for the first few days, and this practice often causes babies to cry. An article in the medical journal *Lancet* concluded that babies who received baths instead of being sponged off retained body heat better, stayed calmer, and did not suffer from any more infections than did babies who got the standard washing treatment. Ask your postpartum nurse how best to care for your baby's navel.

Easing Your Baby's Early Days

Newborn babies show a well-developed sensitivity to pain. Given the standard heel stick to test for jaundice, glucose levels, PKU, and hypothyroidism, a normal newborn tries to withdraw his affected foot and cries. What's more, his heart rate and respiration increase and his blood pressure rises. After being circumcised, male babies will behave differently for at least a day after the surgery.

In the days and weeks that follow the birth, you'll want to know how to minimize such pain for your baby and also how to provide him with comfort when it's needed.

Eye Treatment. Before your baby is released from the delivery area, the routine procedure is for his eyes to be treated with a diluted solution of silver nitrate or an antibiotic ointment. Silver nitrate treatment originated in 1881 in Germany where more than one-third of the childbearing women had incurable gonorrhea. Gonococcal ophthalmia, an eye infection caused by gonorrhea, was then the leading cause of blindness.

Nowadays penicillin, an effective treatment for both gonorrhea and gonococcal ophthalmia, has rendered the universal use of silver nitrate debatable. Alternative treatments, such as erythromycin and tetracycline, have proven as effective as silver nitrate against gonococcal ophthalmia. What's more, these alternative treatments work better than silver nitrate against chlamydial ophthalmia, a venereal infection that is much more prevalent today.

Most hospitals now offer tetracycline or erythromycin as alternatives to silver nitrate treatment. Either antibiotic will be less irritating to your baby's eyes than silver nitrate. But your baby should not get any eye treatment until you have had ample opportunity to examine him and experience the delicious thrill of a wide-eyed mutual gaze. Silver nitrate, particularly, will decrease your baby's visual alertness for the next 48 hours. One mother recalls, "After the eye treatment, Danielle's eyes were swollen shut for several days. We were really happy we'd asked them not to put the drops in for that first hour."

Heel Sticks.   Your baby may get several heel sticks to obtain blood for the diagnosis of several common newborn problems including hypoglycemia and jaundice. Your baby will also be tested for phenylketonuria (PKU) and hypothyroidism. If undetected, these rare disorders could lead to severe mental retardation.

Traditionally, blood is drawn by pricking the baby's heel manually and squeezing until sufficient blood is obtained. Request that the most expert staff member do your baby's heel stick and that your baby be given a pacifier to calm him during the heel-stick procedure. Sucking is a tried and true method of keeping calm for babies who, after all, can't cry and suck at the same time.

Circumcision.   If you have a boy, you will need to decide whether to have him circumcised. In the hospital, your obstetrician or pediatrician performs this surgery, which severs the foreskin of the baby's penis.

In March 1989 the American Academy of Pediatrics (AAP) issued a new statement on circumcision, acknowledging that the procedure has "potential medical benefits and advantages as well as disadvantages and risks. When circumcision is being considered, the benefits and risks should be explained to the parents and informed consent obtained."

AAP's new statement reflected a slight shift from its earlier position, maintained since 1971, that circumcision carried no hygienic or medical advantage. Indeed the academy's earlier indictment of the procedure as of unproven medical worth had driven down the nation's circumcision rates from a high of 95 percent in the 1960s to 58 percent by 1988. In many states, Blue Shield had cut off benefits for the surgery because it was deemed unnecessary.

AAP's cautious about-face followed studies showing that urinary tract infections increased as the circumcision rate fell, and that uncircumcised boys developed more than ten times as many of these potentially life-threatening infections as did circumcised boys.

Critics pointed out that the retrospective studies indicating a rise in urinary tract infections may have been flawed. Indeed, carefully planned prospective studies on circumcision's risks and benefits remain to be done. For this reason, AAP kept its statement clearly noncommittal, emphasizing that parents must weigh what is known about risks and benefits before making their own decision.

In fact, the circumcision issue is hardly clear-cut. Even in uncircumcised babies, urinary tract infections are uncommon. And, while it is true that circumcision in infancy can prevent cancer of the penis, this rare cancer usually occurs only in conditions of poor hygiene exacerbated by sexually transmitted diseases. Cervical cancer is more common among female sexual partners of uncircumcised men infected with papilloma virus, but intercourse at an early age and multiple sex partners pose even greater cancer risks to women. No scientific evidence currently links circumcision status to the incidence of sexually transmitted diseases such as AIDS.

What are the drawbacks of circumcision? First of all, despite popular folklore to the contrary, baby boys *do* respond with pain at having this extremely sensitive part of their bodies cut. Most babies cry and show other physiological changes that indicate they're feeling pain—increased heart rate and agitation during the surgery, for example, and escape into sleep afterwards. Even though the surgery is usually done in the hospital, anesthesia is rarely used.

Several research studies have demonstrated that local anesthetics or nerve blocks reduce babies' pain responses to the surgery without side effects. The American Academy of Pediatrics, however, does not recommend local anesthesia for newborn circumcision. AAP contends that anesthesia adds an element of risk and that data regarding its use have not been reported in a large enough number of cases. A study published in *Pediatrics* in 1991 revealed that sucking on a sucrose-flavored pacifier significantly reduced crying in a group of babies who were being circumcised.

As does any surgery, circumcision includes the risks of pain, hemorrhage, infection, and adhesions. Complications causing serious damage to the penis can occur, but they are exceedingly rare. Of course, circumcision is contraindicated for a sick infant. If your baby is born prematurely, he will not be circumcised before he is ready to be discharged from the hospital.

For some parents, medical risks and benefits are beside the point. In fact, according to several research studies, parents rarely make their decision about circumcision on the basis of medical factors. Instead, a majority of parents choose circumcision for its social or cosmetic benefits. They may want their son to look like his father or like his older brother who was circumcised.

If you're having your baby boy circumcised because of your religious beliefs, the decision will probably be a straightforward one for you. The benefits of your son's circumcision stem from the communal ritual observance of an age-old ceremony. In your case, these benefits will probably outweigh the drawbacks of elective surgery.

In a Jewish ritual circumcision performed by a *mohel,* your baby probably will not receive local anesthesia unless you arrange to have a doctor present as well. An occasional *mohel* uses a topical anesthetic spray, but traditionally, the *Brit Milah* or *Bris* is performed with the baby sucking on a small gauze pad soaked in sweet ceremonial wine. The alcohol isn't sufficient to provide analgesia, but the action of sucking can calm your baby as he undergoes the stress of being circumcised.

Should you decide not to circumcise your son, rest assured that teaching a little boy to keep his uncircumcised penis clean is about as hard as teaching him to clean his ears. That is to say, it requires some teaching but it can be done (see Resources for information on caring for an uncircumcised boy).

Everyday Aches and Pains

Crying is your baby's first form of communication. When he cries, he's using the only way he knows to tell you he needs something. Styles in baby care change. Parents used to be told that if they responded to their babies' cries, the babies would cry more. But research suggests that it's actually just the opposite: the more rapidly and appropriately you address your baby's needs, the less your baby will cry.

Whole books have been written about infant crying and what to do about it. It's a fact that some babies really do cry more than others, and that for the first three months of your baby's life you can expect to hear *a lot* of crying. But it still helps to know the most effective ways of soothing your baby's discomfort.

If hunger's not the problem—and it often is—try holding your baby close to you so he can feel your warmth. Your baby's skin is his largest sense organ; this makes touch a tremendously important comfort for him. Parents all over the world lift, hold, stroke, rock, and walk their crying babies. A rocking chair will soothe both you and your baby.

Many parents like to use the soft fabric carriers that enable them to hold their baby close but still give them the luxury of having their hands free (see Resources). When your baby is snuggled against your chest, he can feel your warmth, smell your familiar scent, and hear your heartbeat. In fact, a study by Dr. Urs A. Hunziker and Dr. Ronald G. Barr demonstrated that infants who were carried for about two hours extra each day in addition to the normal holding for feedings and comfort cried much less in the first three months of life than did infants who were not given the extra comfort.

Babies like slow, smooth, rhythmic motion whether or not they're being held, so you may want to consider using a cradle, wind-up swing, or crib hammock to keep your baby happy. You may also like to introduce your baby to a pacifier. Sucking is one of your baby's primary needs and it's a natural soother for a baby in distress. But use a pacifier only if your baby's weight gain is good. The pacifier should never become a substitute for needed food.

For several months, your baby won't understand any of the words you say. But the way you meet your baby's basic needs for sleep, warmth, food, and solace will eloquently express your love for him in the only language he can yet comprehend.

20
Easing Pain in the Immediate Postpartum

Your body underwent tremendous change throughout the nine months preceding the birth; amazingly, in just six weeks afterwards your organs will return to their original condition. Many of the transformations take place quite automatically. Others will require some effort on your part, and a few may cause you some discomfort.

Afterpains. You'll know your body is working hard to get back into shape by the presence of uterine contractions, often called "afterpains," after the birth. These contractions serve the important function of clamping off open blood vessels at the placental site, minimizing your loss of blood after giving birth. If your uterus doesn't contract well after the baby is born, you may be given Pitocin to aid the process—many doctors routinely add Pitocin to your IV—and a labor and delivery nurse will firmly massage the fundus or top of your uterus every so often to make sure that it stays contracted.

If you're planning to breastfeed, see if your baby will latch on shortly after the delivery. He's apt to be more wide awake then than he'll be for the next few days. What's more, the stimulation of your nipples promotes oxytocin secretion which keeps your uterus contracted.

First-time mothers don't usually find the postpartum uterine con-tractions as painful as do second-timers. Whether it is your first or a subsequent birth, concentrate on breathing and relaxing when the nurse does the fundal massage because this procedure may prompt more painful contractions. You may find it less painful to do your own massage; ask the nurse to show you how.

If you've given birth before, your after-contractions may be quite painful for about 24 hours after the birth, particularly when you're nursing your baby. "I found it very helpful to do slow, relaxed breathing while nursing the baby," one mother says.

An occasional first-time mother finds her afterpains exceedingly painful. One new mother recalls, "The contractions were so strong my legs would shake and I felt nauseous. Since I didn't have an epi-siotomy, that was really the only discomfort I felt after the birth." You should be aware that persistent severe cramps or uterine tender-ness could be a sign of infection. To relieve the pain of after-contrac-tions, try spending some time lying on your abdomen. If your afterpains are especially uncomfortable, you could also apply a heat-ing pad to your abdomen or take a mild painkiller such as aceta-minophen. To minimize the passage of drugs in your breast milk, it's best to take painkillers either right before or right after breastfeeding.

You may find herbal remedies effective. Robin Lim, author of *After the Baby's Birth*, suggests the following teas, available at many health food stores, as effective in relieving the pain of postpartum contractions: motherwort, shepherd's purse, and false unicorn.

Urinating.   Shortly after the birth, you'll be asked to urinate, and this can really sting. It's crucial to keep your bladder empty, though, because a full bladder makes the afterpains feel a lot worse. It may help to put some warm water on your perineum. Most hospitals give you a little plastic "peri-care" bottle to squirt water on yourself after toileting. You can use this squeeze bottle to encourage the flow of urine as you sit on the toilet. Drinking a lot dilutes the acidity of your urine and helps lessen the stinging sensation. Be prepared to urinate (and sweat) much more than usual in the next few days. Your body needs to get rid of all the extra fluids you held during pregnancy to maintain a greatly increased blood volume.

Bowel Movements.   It's perfectly normal not to have to move your bowels for a few days after delivery. You probably had diarrhea or an enema and you haven't eaten much for a while. For your own comfort, pay special attention to keeping your stools soft. Emphasize high-fiber foods like fruits, vegetables, and whole grains, and drink plenty of liquids to soften your stools and minimize the amount of straining necessary to move your bowels. Prunes or prune juice, and bran (available in health food stores) are popular natural laxatives. Walking also helps to promote your normal bowel function. Let your doctor or midwife know if you haven't moved your bowels within a week.

Episiotomy.   The stitches from your episiotomy may be the most uncomfortable part of your postpartum. Nowadays, it's common treatment to receive an ice pack on the perineum for the first 12 to 24 hours, followed by encouragement to take plenty of warm sitz baths.

One mother says, "For anyone who dreads an episiotomy—I certainly did—and ends up having one—maybe you'll have a nine-pound-eleven-ounce kid in a hurry like I did—I highly recommend the ice packs and begged the nurses for a new one practically every two hours. After the first day of relative discomfort, I healed rapidly and felt completely back to normal within the week."

You may take the portable sitz bath home from the hospital with you or you can buy a sitz bath at a pharmacy for soaks after you go home. If you soak in your own bathtub, make sure it's clean, wash your feet before getting in, and keep the water depth under four inches.

Some doctors disagree with the advice to switch to warm sitz baths after 24 hours. Dr. William Droegemueller, professor of obstetrics and gynecology at the University of North Carolina, advocates ice-cold sitz baths for the duration of episiotomy pain. He points out that, for athletic injuries, ice baths have long been substituted for hot whirlpools. According to Droegemueller, perineal injuries should be treated the same way because ice treatment reduces the swelling, muscle irritability, and spasm that cause most of the pain from an injury.

Of course, it sounds quite unappealing to lower your bottom into a tub of ice water. But after you get past the initial discomfort of the burning, icy sensation, you can obtain good pain relief for four to six hours afterwards. In Droegemueller's study, patients who alternated between hot and cold sitz baths preferred the cold baths for extended pain relief. In contrast, a warm sitz bath feels good as long as you're sitting in it, but 30 minutes after getting out, you may be increasingly aware of perineal pain.

If you decide to try an ice bath, sit in tap water to which ice is added. The faster the water temperature is lowered, the shorter the uncomfortable period will last. Ideally, you should stay in the ice bath for twenty to thirty minutes. Do the pelvic floor contractions (Kegel exercises), which you learned in your childbirth class, during the last few minutes of the bath.

To do the Kegel exercise, tighten the muscles around your vagina and urethra as though you were trying to interrupt the flow of urine. Hold for about ten seconds and release. Repeat four times. Do this exercise in sets of five ten-second contractions at least ten times each day.

In addition to doing the Kegel exercise in your sitz bath and regularly throughout the day, contract your pelvic floor muscles before you stand, sit, or do any activity that puts stress on these muscles. Other aids to healing your episiotomy are walking and applying witch hazel compresses to your perineum.

Hemorrhoids.   If you've had hemorrhoids during pregnancy or perhaps pushed them out at birth, you know how annoying they can be. Fortunately, they eventually do recede after birth. Ice packs and cold sitz baths will help shrink your hemorrhoids. Witch hazel compresses can also be soothing. After you use the toilet, replace your hemorrhoids with your finger using a finger cot—available in the hospital— or just some toilet paper lubricated with vaseline. Lying prone with your hips elevated on a pillow will also encourage your hemorrhoids to recede back into your anus.

The doughnut cushion which is sometimes given to you to aid sitting on your episiotomy stitches can actually exacerbate hemorrhoids. If you can, it's preferable to replace your hemorrhoids in your anus, contract your pelvic floor muscles, and sit on a firm surface. You may find it easier to sit tilted to one side or the other, rather than putting all your weight on your perineum.

After a Cesarean.   If your baby is born by cesarean, you'll be recovering from major surgery as well as from childbirth. Your skin incision will be tender and it will hurt to use the muscles which have been cut.

After any surgery, it's important to try to get your body moving again, so wiggle your toes around and rotate your ankles as soon as you get feeling back in your legs. The nurses will teach you to deep-breathe, and to cough or huff in order to clear your lungs. Walking as soon as possible after the surgery helps to prevent blood clots and will reduce the gas pains that signal that your intestines are back in working condition.

These gas pains may be intensely uncomfortable. The following exercise to prevent or ease gas pains is adapted from "Cesarean Birth—A Special Delivery" by Marianne Brorup-Weston and Penny Simkin, a pamphlet which may be ordered from Pennypress (see Resources):

Frequently during the first five postpartum days, place both hands or a pillow on your incision. Take a deep breath in, allowing your abdomen to expand. Let your breath out slowly, pulling your abdominal muscles in.

Rocking in a rocking chair three or four times a day for a total of about an hour may also ease post-cesarean gas pains. Put pillows under your feet to spare your sore abdominal muscles.

The most uncomfortable times after a cesarean are fundal massage, changing positions, walking, and coughing. Whenever possible, splint your incision with your hands to make these activities less uncomfortable. If you need pain medications, take them before you're in intense pain, preferably about a half hour before you anticipate an uncomfortable activity. Breastfeeding your baby with a pillow on your abdomen or holding him in the football hold, under your arm, can also spare pain to your incision.

Transcutaneous electrical nerve stimulation (TENS), occasionally used to alleviate labor pain (see chapter 7), also offers many benefits to the woman who is recovering from a cesarean delivery. Russell Foley, TENS expert, comments, "Taking patients' pain away with TENS gives them better mobility, and that's important because the most traumatic thing to the body after an operation is immobilization. The longer a person is immobilized, the harder it is to recover."

Using TENS can mean you'll need fewer narcotic painkillers after your surgery. Indeed, a study published in *Physical Therapy* in 1986 showed that women who used TENS following cesarean birth used significantly less Demerol for pain relief. Narcotics such as Demerol, says Russell Foley, "suppress gastrointestinal motility, change respiration, and alter heart rate. If you remove the need for medication by using TENS, you can also remove the side effects of medications."

If you use TENS for your post-cesarean recovery, the electrodes can be positioned immediately after suturing, and taped to your abdomen under the dressing. You'll be taught to use the monitor in order to control the amount of electrical stimulation you receive. The monitor can be detached so that you can shower normally. TENS is usually used just for the first two post-cesarean days.

Many hospitals employ patient-controlled analgesia (PCA), an intravenous system that enables postoperative patients to control their own pain relief after surgery. A study of post-cesarean patients published in *Obstetrics and Gynecology* revealed that women using PCA experienced fewer side effects and got more dependable relief than women who had to depend on the nurses for intermittent pain injections. The typical patient uses PCA for just 24 hours after surgery.

Once your outside stitches are removed (occasionally these aren't stitches but rather staples or clamps), you'll return home, usually within three days to five days. Regardless of how well you feel, it's important to take your recovery slowly. Avoid heavy lifting for six weeks, and see if you can secure outside help for the necessary household tasks.

Breastfeeding

Breastfeeding is the most natural way to feed your baby an ideal food. Not only does the process of breastfeeding bring you closer to your baby, it's usually a pleasurable experience for both of you. In addition, nursing promotes your body's recovery after you've given birth.

If you plan to breastfeed, the first thing you should do is get a good basic resource book on nursing, such as *The Nursing Mother's Companion* by Kathleen Huggins. You should also identify a support person who has had a happy nursing experience. This may be a friend, sister, La Leche League leader, lactation consultant, childbirth educator, midwife, nurse, or doctor. It's vitally important to have someone who can tell you, "Yes, that happened to me; I lived through it and so can you." You'll also need to enlist the wholehearted support of your husband, as well as that of your obstetrician or midwife and your baby's doctor.

The doctor who takes care of your baby can be a great help to breastfeeding or a major stumbling block. You'll rarely speak to a doctor who is openly hostile about breastfeeding, but "most of them just give lip service to it," says Dr. Jay N. Gordon, a medical consultant to La Leche League and a pediatrician in Santa Monica, California. To find a doctor who is truly supportive of breastfeeding, ask your prospective doctor how many of his or her patients nurse; how long mothers usually nurse; what the doctor recommends if breastfeeding problems arise; when the doctor advocates introducing solid foods; and why and how the doctor might suggest weaning.

Sometimes problems arise which may make you wonder whether it's really worth it to keep nursing your baby. Rest assured that it definitely is worth it. When you have correct information and strong emotional support, you'll find most nursing problems to be preventable, or temporary and easily solved.

For example, engorgement and sore nipples—two of the commonest problems for new nursing mothers—can be prevented or cured by feeding your new baby as soon as possible after the birth, feeding as frequently as possible thereafter, and making sure your baby is correctly positioned on your breast.

To position your baby, hold him facing your chest. You may want to put a pillow on your lap to support the baby so that you don't get a backache. With your opposite hand, hold your breast with your thumb and fingers describing a C-shape around the areola or colored portion. Tickle your baby's lips gently with your nipple, and, when he opens his mouth wide, center your nipple and some of the areola into his mouth. Hold him close enough so that he is able to compress the areola with his jaws rather than just hanging on to the edge of the nipple (which would make you *very* sore). If necessary, depress an air passage for him by pressing down on your breast with your thumb.

Engorgement.   Engorgement, the swelling that frequently occurs on about the second or third day, poses much less of a problem if you nurse your baby on demand from birth on. Rigidly scheduled feedings tend to exacerbate the problem because when your breasts get too full, the pain that results can inhibit your ability to "let down" the milk so your baby can get it. Engorgement also makes it hard for the baby to grasp the nipple properly, so he gums it instead. This causes even more soreness.

If you become engorged, remember that it's a temporary condition. You can get some relief by standing in a shower facing away from the flow of water. Allow the warm water to flow over your shoulders onto your breasts, and hand express some milk. Warm compresses applied before a feeding achieve the same effect. If your nipple and areola are rigid, preventing your baby from latching on properly, be sure to express a little milk before each feeding to soften the nipple so that the baby can get it to the back of his mouth.

Sore nipples.   Sore nipples commonly accompany the early days of nursing. Contrary to popular advice, buffing your nipples with a terry cloth towel prior to delivery is not a good way to get your nipples ready for nursing. Pressure, not friction, is what you'll be experiencing with breastfeeding, so your husband's caresses and kisses will probably be much more effective—and more fun too!

Actually, prenatal nipple preparation is not really necessary. It's more important just to avoid irritating your nipples. Don't wash them with soap or any other drying agent, and don't even wash them with water too vigorously as this reduces natural lubricants. To avoid sore nipples, position your baby correctly at your breast and take care to release the suction at the end of a feeding by inserting a little finger into the baby's mouth rather than pulling the baby off the breast abruptly.

Nurses used to think—some still do—that sore nipples could be prevented by limiting sucking time and spacing the nursings at wide intervals. Many studies have shown that this treatment merely postpones nipple soreness. Limiting sucking time also deprives the baby of the rich and nutritious milk that only emerges toward the end of a feeding. As far as nipple soreness is concerned, spacing the feedings can actually make matters worse by creating a ravenous baby who latches on with a vengeance that really hurts! What's more, spacing the feedings promotes the very engorgement that leads to sore nipples.

Feeding your baby on demand—early and often—seems to be the best policy. As long as he is positioned correctly, it doesn't seem to matter how long each feeding takes. In general, it's better to watch your baby than it is to watch the clock.

If your nipples get sore, you may temporarily want to confine the feedings on the sore side to five minutes. Until you feel better, start each feeding on the least sore side, because it's the first minute of each feeding that is usually the most painful. Since the primary stress on your nipple comes from the baby's tongue, vary the position of the baby's mouth on your nipple by using alternative feeding positions like the football hold described above.

You can leave some milk on your nipple after the feeding because breast milk helps to heal sore nipples. Then try to air dry your nipples for ten to 15 minutes. Sunlight speeds the healing process, as does a hair dryer set on low.

As peculiar as it sounds, a tea strainer placed over your nipple inside your bra will allow air to circulate and promote healing. There are also special shields designed for this purpose. Another kind of shield can draw out a flat or inverted nipple. Consult a local La Leche League leader if you need advice on where to obtain nipple shields for either of these problems.

Some women find it helps to apply ice or cold water before a feeding to make their nipples more erect and easier for the baby to grasp without gumming.

A healthy nipple needs no artificial lubrication. But if your nipples become dry from too-vigorous nursing, you may wish to apply a tiny amount of lubricant for your own comfort. Choose a lubricant you don't need to wash off before the next feeding and use it sparingly around the nipple only.

A light vegetable oil, such as canola, safflower, or sunflower, may be your best choice. Alcohol-based products such as commercial breast creams will only dry your nipples. Products containing lanolin, vitamin E, or cocoa butter may trigger an allergic reaction. You should also avoid petroleum products, such as baby oil, petroleum jelly, or A and D ointment, and heavy oils such as olive or peanut oil. These lubricants prevent air from reaching your skin. Before you apply any oil, make sure your nipples are completely dry after a feeding.

The nipple shields commonly offered in the hospital to alleviate sore nipples and feeding problems should be avoided if possible. Because the shields contain only one hole, the baby needs to nurse longer to get the same amount of milk. Prolonged use can actually decrease your milk supply. If you decide to use the shield, remove it as soon as the baby draws your nipple out, within the first minute or so of the feeding. Every day, cut away a little more of the shield, starting at the center and working out, to maximize the necessary contact of the baby's mouth to your nipple.

Pads to control milk leakage should be cotton, not plastic, which holds in the moisture. Use all-cotton bras and wash them in mild detergents that don't leave irritating residues. Remember that sore nipples are very common but very temporary.

Breast Infections.   A high fever along with hardening and tenderness of your breast can signal a breast infection. Breast infections are thought to be caused by incomplete drainage of your breast, occasionally promoted by engorgement or by a too-tight bra which may plug a duct and impede the milk flow. To treat a breast infection, call your doctor and remember this simple rule: "Heat, rest, and empty breast." In other words, apply hot compresses, take the baby to bed with you, and keep on nursing.

Your doctor probably will prescribe an antibiotic, which should not affect your milk. The baby will receive antibodies to the infection as he nurses. It's very important to take the antibiotic for the full ten days even though you'll probably feel better within a few days.

Bottle Feeding

If you're planning to bottle feed your baby, you should expect to suffer temporarily from painful engorgement of your breasts. The chemical treatments commonly used to suppress lactation may merely postpone the engorgement process rather than prevent it.

Milk-suppressing drugs are of two types: hormonal treatments, such as Tace and Deladumone, and a prolactin inhibitor, Parlodel. Hormonal treatment for milk inhibition has been associated with an increased risk of blood clots. Parlodel's potential side effects may be more annoying than life-threatening: lowered blood pressure, nausea, headaches, and dizziness. If you do use any of these drugs, you should start on the first postpartum day and you'll need to take the medication for 14 days.

To stop your milk production naturally, you can simply use ice packs and binding. Ice packs numb the breasts and constrict blood vessels, thereby alleviating one cause of engorgement. A tight bra or binder decreases your milk supply, taking care of the other cause of engorgement. Start this treatment shortly after delivery and continue it for five days. You may also want to use aspirin or acetaminophen for the pain of engorgement, which peaks on the third or fourth day and rarely lasts more than a day or two. Be sure to avoid putting warm water on your breasts or emptying your breasts by squeezing your nipples, because these actions will only stimulate your milk production.

Going Home

After you go home from the hospital, it's especially important to take good care of yourself. The fact that you have enormous new responsibilities makes this more difficult, of course, but it's all the more necessary to meet your needs for rest and nourishment. As discussed in chapter 2, the myth of the primitive woman who gives birth and then keeps on working in the field is just that: a myth. In almost every society in the world, a woman who has just given birth gets an extended rest period afterwards.

Now that women are going home from the hospital an average of two days after a vaginal delivery, new-parent care services have proliferated all over the country. The National Association of Postpartum Care Services (NAPCS), a clearinghouse for such programs, boasts more than 80 members across the country with names like New Mother's Home Companion in Madison, Wisconsin, Mother-Care Services in Lenox, Massachusetts, Motherlove in Indianapolis, Indiana, and Mothering Mom in Liverpool, New York. Nationally, costs range from about $10 to more than $30 per hour. The more hours a new mother signs up for, the lower the cost.

The Mother's Cradle in Chicago is typical of these postpartum programs. Marilyn Kearns Davis, president of Mother's Cradle, says, "We nurture the new mom during the transition time after childbirth. We've trained five doulas, all but one of them mothers themselves, and new mothers can sign up for a variety of different packages. The most popular package is 48 hours for $575. Typically, the doula will go into the home, see if the mother needs help with the baby, answer any questions, prepare lunch, and encourage the mother to rest. We also offer breastfeeding support."

If you cannot afford or prefer not to hire a postpartum helper, you may want at least to hire out some of the essential household tasks such as grocery shopping and housecleaning for a few weeks. Rest is a precious commodity when you have a brand-new baby to take care of. Here are a few more suggestions:

- Lower your expectations of what you can accomplish.
- Keep housework to a bare minimum.
- Simplify with the use of frozen meals, casseroles from friends, paper plates, etc.
- Discourage visitors but make sure everyone who comes pitches in by providing a meal and helping out with the housework.
- Sleep whenever the baby naps.
- Unplug your phone when you go to sleep.
- Try to obtain sitters early and remember to take time for yourself.

Sex.   For a while after the birth, resuming your sexual relationship with your husband may be the last thing on your mind. Fatigue, the vast new responsibility of the baby, and the immense hormonal shifts of the birth can all temporarily reduce your sex drive. It's especially important to communicate with your partner so that you can fulfill each other's needs for closeness—perhaps for a time by kissing, touching, and massage rather than intercourse.

Once the bright red vaginal bleeding known as lochia has stopped, you can safely resume sexual relations. This may be after only a week or so, but you should wait until you're emotionally as well as physically ready for sex. As one obstetrician puts it, "If it feels good, do it, but if it hurts, don't do it."

Your first intercourse may or may not be painful. A dry "tight" feeling may be due to your episiotomy stitches or to the lack of vaginal lubrication, which is especially common if you are nursing. K-Y jelly, a water-soluble lubricant available without prescription at your drugstore, can provide some lubrication so you don't "squeak" when you make love.

Try a hot bath to relax yourself prior to intercourse, and experiment with positions that take some of the stress off your stitches. Making love side by side, with the woman on top, or with the husband entering from the rear will probably all feel more comfortable to you than the "missionary" position.

Actually, lovemaking helps to heal your perineum and can soften your scar if you've had stitches. Sex may not feel terrific the first time or even the first few times, but it should get better. If pain persists, be sure to consult your doctor or midwife. Rest assured that your normal sexual feelings will come back. But for a time, being absorbed in caring for a new baby can quite normally supersede just about everything else in your life.

General Care

While this chapter has focused on very specific aches and pains, you may not experience anything so specialized, yet you still may not feel quite "yourself" for some time after giving birth. The changes of new motherhood are psychological as well as physical, so be extra patient with yourself.

Because you're giving so much to the baby, you should concentrate on getting postpartum care that nourishes you. It's crucial, of course, to eat well, to get enough rest, and to revitalize yourself with exercise. Ask your childbirth educator for exercises that are most appropriate for the first few days and weeks after your baby's birth. Within about two or three weeks after an uncomplicated birth, you can enroll in an exercise class specifically oriented to postpartum mothers.

Some of the techniques that helped you during labor may come in handy after the baby is born, too. For example, if you can afford it, treat yourself to a professional massage. This feels good anytime, but it is exceptionally valuable now. Acupuncture, too, offers traditional treatments after the birth of a child. These treatments can enhance your milk production, encourage the healing of your episiotomy or cesarean incision, and generally make you feel revitalized. Many women use visualization and/or hypnotic techniques to promote their postpartum recovery. The breathing and relaxation techniques you used for labor can also come in handy during the challenging early days of parenting.

Remember that taking good care of your baby requires taking good care of yourself, too. If you pay adequate attention to your own needs, you'll be better able to enjoy caring for your new baby.

21
Making Your Own
Best Choices

After reading this book, you may feel as though you'd need a U-Haul to carry all the necessities to the hospital with you! Actually, much more important than what you bring with you is the careful groundwork you'll lay in preparation for giving birth. No one, of course, could possibly do all the things suggested in this book. However, as you've been reading, you probably found that certain methods of pain relief seemed particularly appealing. Using the Resources section at the end of this book, pursue the avenues that make the most sense to you. The following paragraphs may provide a rough timetable for you to follow.

As soon as possible in pregnancy, research your options for childbirth and new-baby care. Explore your preferences with prospective birth attendants and tour different hospitals and birthing centers to discover if they meet your individual needs. Make an early reservation for the type of childbirth preparation class that appeals most to you. If possible, take an early pregnancy class which will teach you about exercise and nutrition appropriate for pregnancy. Some women will want to consult an acupuncturist, hypnotherapist, or biofeedback specialist for pregnancy problems such as high blood pressure, nausea, or headaches.

During the middle months of pregnancy, research the feasibility of having a female labor companion and begin to practice the relaxation techniques found in chapter 4. This is a good time to begin getting regularly massaged, either by your husband or by a professional massage therapist. If you plan to use hypnosis, acupuncture, TENS, or biofeedback to help you relax in labor, you should make arrangements with the appropriate professionals at this stage of pregnancy.

During the final trimester of your pregnancy, you'll probably be taking childbirth classes and practicing the breathing, relaxation, and visualization techniques discussed earlier. Begin accumulating your bag of goodies to take to the hospital with you, and select the music you'd like to play during labor.

Toward the end of pregnancy is also a good time to discuss your preferences and questions about labor and delivery medications with your birth attendant, and to make final plans for the birth and immediate postpartum. It's particularly helpful to write up a birth plan and bring it to the hospital with you, especially if your attendant practices with a large group of doctors or midwives. The plan should include your preferences for an "ideal" delivery as well as for a difficult one, and should recognize the need for flexibility if the medical situation warrants a change in procedures.

Include in your plan all the elements that are most important to you for the birth, and discuss it with your birth attendant several weeks in advance of your due date. An excellent pamphlet which discusses the use of a birth plan and includes a sample plan with many options can be ordered from Pennypress, Inc. (see Resources). Particularly if you're planning to do something different from the normal hospital routine, it's essential to plan it out in advance, making sure that you have your birth attendant's cooperation.

One of my students wrote the following plan. Its language indicated her flexibility and her willingness to cooperate fully with the medical personnel who attended her:

> If at all possible, we would prefer the following treatment during labor, delivery, and recovery. We understand, however, that medical conditions at the time might necessitate alternative treatment.
>
> 1. Birthing room: The doctor has approved our use of the birthing room.
>
> 2. Episiotomy: We have started to massage my perineum. If at all possible, we would like to avoid an episiotomy, but would understand if conditions dictate otherwise.
>
> 3. Delivery: We would prefer that the baby be placed on my abdomen soon after birth and that she remain with us through the recovery period.

4. Eyedrops: We would prefer to use erythromycin and that the eyedrops not be instilled until one hour after birth so that the baby can see clearly during that first hour.

5. Sugar water/artificial nipples: We understand that the baby must be in the nursery for four hours of observation. During this time we would prefer that she not be given sugar water unless medically indicated, or any artificial nipples. If she awakes and needs to be fed, please bring her to me for breastfeeding.

6. Rooming-in: At this point we would prefer 24-hour rooming in. Needless to say, our final decision will be based on the condition of mother and child.

Thank you very much for your consideration of our requests.

The creation of this type of plan—substituting, of course, the things that are most important to you—will help you to think more clearly about your goals for the delivery. Secure in the confidence that you've done everything within your power to make this the very best experience possible, you'll be able to yield fully to the exciting challenge of giving birth.

Resources

ACUPUNCTURE

American Association for
Acupuncture and Oriental
Medicine
1424 16th St. NW, Suite 501
Washington, DC 20036
(202) 265-2287

Call or write to get a local referral.

Acupuncture Research Institute
313 W. Andrix St.
Monterey Park, CA 91754
(213) 722-7353

ALTERNATIVE BIRTHING CENTERS

National Association of
Childbearing Centers
3123 Gottschall Rd.
Perkiomenville, PA 18074-9546
(215) 234-8068
(215) 234-0564 (FAX)

Send SASE and $1 to cover cost of
mailings.

National Association of Parents
and Professionals for Safe
Alternatives in Childbirth
(NAPSAC, International)
Rt. 1, Box 646
Marble Hill, MO 63764-9726
(314) 238-2010

BABY CARRIERS

NoJo
22942 Arroyo Vista
Rancho Santa Margareta, CA
92688
(800) 541-5711

The Right Start Catalog
Right Start Plaza
5334 Sterling Center Dr.
Westlake Village, CA 91361

BIOFEEDBACK

Association for Applied
Psychophysiology and
Biofeedback
10200 W. 44th Ave., Suite 304
Wheat Ridge, CO 80033
(303) 422-8436

Send SASE.

Stress Dots:

Shirley Stokoe and Associates
Choices Through Communication
1333 West 120th Ave., Suite 110
Westminster, CO 80234
(303) 450-2787

Biodots:
ICEA Bookcenter
P.O. Box 20048
Minneapolis, MN 55420

BIRTHING BEDS

ARJO-Century, Inc.
6380 Oakton St.
Morton Grove, IL 60053
(708) 967-0360

Hill-Rom
Highway 46
Batesville, IN 47006
(800) 445-3730

BREASTFEEDING INFORMATION

Childbirth Graphics Ltd.
P.O. Box 20540
Rochester, NY 14602-0540
(716) 272-0300

International Lactation Consultant
  Association
201 Brown Ave.
Evanston, IL 60202
(708) 260-8874

Health Education Associates, Inc.
8 Jan Sebastian Way, Unit 13
Sandwich, MA 02563
(508) 888-8044

La Leche League International
9616 Minneapolis Ave.
Franklin Park, IL 60130-8209
(312) 455-7730
(800) LA-LECHE

Check your White Pages for local
listing.

CESAREAN DELIVERY, CESAREAN PREVENTION, AND
VAGINAL BIRTH AFTER CESAREAN

C/SEC, Inc.
22 Forest Rd.
Framingham, MA 01701
(617) 877-8266

Cesarean Prevention Movement
P.O. Box 152, University Station
Syracuse, NY 13210
(315) 424-1942

Pamphlets on cesarean birth and on vaginal birth after cesarean can be
ordered from Pennypress (see Mail-Order section, below).

CHILDBIRTH EDUCATION

American Academy of Husband-
  Coached Childbirth
  (The Bradley Method)
P.O. Box 5224
Sherman Oaks, CA 91413
(818) 788-6662
(800) 423-2397

The Council of Childbirth
  Education Specialists, Inc.
8 Sylvan Glen
East Lyme, CT 06333
(203) 739-8912

Training for labor and delivery
nurses.

American Society for
  Psychoprophylaxis in Obstetrics
  (ASPO/Lamaze)
1101 Connecticut Ave. NW
Washington, DC 20036
(800) 368-4404

Gamper International, Inc.
  (formerly Midwest Parentcraft
  Center)
627 Beaver Rd.
Glenview, IL 60025

CHILDBIRTH EDUCATION
(Continued)

Informed Homebirth/Informed
  Birth and Parenting
P.O. Box 3675
Ann Arbor, MI 48106
(313) 662-6857

International Childbirth Education
  Association (ICEA)
P.O. Box 20048
Minneapolis, MN 55420-0048
(612) 854-8660

Positive Pregnancy and Parenting
  Fitness (Yoga)
Sylvia Klein Olkin, M.S.
51 Saltrock Rd.
Baltic, CT 06330
(203) 822-8573
(800) 433-5523

Read Natural Childbirth
  Foundation, Inc.
P.O. Box 150956
San Rafael, CA 94915
(415) 456-8462

CIRCUMCISION

National Organization of
  Circumcision Information
  Resource Centers (NOCIRC)
P.O. Box 2512
San Anselmo, CA 94979-2512
(415) 488-9883

Pamphlets on circumcision and on the care of an uncircumcised boy can be
ordered from Pennypress (see Mail-Order section, below).

COMFORT MEASURES FOR LABOR

Expectancy Resources
317 S. Delmar
Decatur, IL 62522
(217) 423-6022

Offers fan with printed list of
comfort measures for labor; also
available in Spanish.

EXERCISE

The American College of
   Obstetricians and Gynecologists
   (ACOG)
Resource Center
409 12th St. SW
Washington, DC 20024

Send SASE to receive pamphlet,
"Exercise and Fitness: A Guide for
Women."

Stretching, Inc.
P.O. Box 767
Palmer Lake, CO 80133
(719) 481-3928
(800) 333-1307

"Pregnancy Stretches," a laminated
one-sheet summary of stretching
exercises, is available for $2 plus
$1.75 shipping.

Prenatal exercise videotapes are available from many mail-order catalogs
(see Mail-Order section, below), or from the following two sources:

Elize St. Charles and Associates
20409 Old Santa Cruz Highway
Los Gatos, CA 95030
(800) 452-4466

People in Motion, Inc.
1395 Fawnwood Dr.
Monument, CO 80132
(719) 481-3565
(800) 937-7733 for charge card
   orders.

HOME BIRTH

Association for Childbirth at
   Home International (ACHI)
Box 430
Glendale, CA 91209
(213) 667-0839
(818) 545-7128

National Association of Parents
   and Professionals for Safe
   Alternatives in Childbirth
   (NAPSAC, International)
Rt. 1, Box 646
Marble Hill, MO 63764-9726
(314) 238-2010

Informed Homebirth/Informed
   Birth and Parenting
P.O. Box 3675
Ann Arbor, MI 48106
(313) 662-6857

HOT AND COLD PACKS

COLPAC
Chattanooga Group, Inc.
4717 Adams Rd.
P.O. Box 489
Hixson, TN 37343

Reusable cold products.

3M ColdHot Pack
Medical Division
3M Health Care
3M Center Bldg. 225-5S-01
St. Paul, MN 55144-1000
(800) 228-3957

Reusable hot and cold pack.

HYPNOSIS

American Society of Clinical
   Hypnosis
2200 E. Devon, Suite 291
Des Plaines, IL 60018
(708) 297-3317

Send SASE.

Society for Clinical and
   Experimental Hypnosis
128-A Kings Park Dr.
Liverpool, NY 13090
(315) 652-7299

Send SASE.

LABOR SUPPORT

Informed Homebirth/Informed
   Birth and Parenting
P.O. Box 3675
Ann Arbor, MI 48106
(313) 662-6857

International Childbirth Education
   Association (ICEA)
P.O. Box 20048
Minneapolis, MN 55420-0048
(612) 854-8660

National Association of Childbirth
   Assistants (NACA)
Claudia Lowe, Director
P.O. Box 12037
Santa Rosa, CA 95043
(408) 225-9167

A pamphlet on labor support can be ordered from Pennypress (see Mail-
Order section, below).

MAIL-ORDER BOOKS, PAMPHLETS, AUDIOCASSETTES AND VIDEOCASSETTES ON BIRTH AND PARENTING

Call or write for current catalog:

ASPO/Lamaze of Los Angeles, Inc.
2931 S. Sepulveda Blvd., Suite F
Los Angeles, CA 90064-3912
(310) 479-8669

National bookstore for ASPO/
Lamaze.

Be Healthy, Inc.
The Specialty Catalog for
   Expectant and New Parents
51 Saltrock Rd.
Baltic, CT 06330
(203) 822-8573
(800) 433-5523

Birth and Life Bookstore
P.O. Box 70625
Seattle, WA 98107-0625
(206) 789-4444

Childbirth Graphics Ltd.
P.O. Box 20540
Rochester, NY 14602-0540
(716) 272-0300

Health Education Associates, Inc.
8 Jan Sebastian Way, Unit 13
Sandwich, MA 02563
(508) 888-8044

MAIL-ORDER BOOKS, PAMPHLETS, AUDIOCASSETTES AND VIDEOCASSETTES ON BIRTH AND PARENTING
(Continued)

ICEA Bookcenter
P.O. Box 20048
Minneapolis, MN 55420
(612) 854-8660

Informed Homebirth/Informed
Birth and Parenting
P.O. Box 3675
Ann Arbor, MI 48106
(313) 662-6857

Injoy Productions
(Videotapes only)
1490 Riverside Ave.
Boulder, CO 80304
(303) 447-2082

Pennypress
1100 23rd Ave. E.
Seattle, WA 98112
(206) 325-1419

MASSAGE

American Massage Therapy
Association
1130 W. North Shore Ave.
Chicago, IL 60626-4670
(312) 761-2682

Stretching, Inc.
P.O. Box 767
Palmer Lake, CO 80133
(719) 481-3928
(800) 333-1307

Offers a variety of body tools for massage or self-massage.

MIDWIVES

American College of Nurse-
Midwives (ACNM)
1522 K St. NW, Suite 1000
Washington, DC 20005
(202) 289-0171

Midwives' Alliance of North
America (MANA)
P.O. Box 1121
Bristol, VA 24203
(615) 764-5561

MUSIC FOR RELAXATION

Gateways Institute
P.O. Box 1778
Ojai, CA 93024
(800) 777-8908

Hearts of Space
P.O. Box 31321
San Francisco, CA 94131
(415) 759-1130

National Association for Music
Therapy
8455 Colesville Rd., Suite 930
Silver Spring, MD 20910
(301) 589-3300

Send SASE.

Sound Rx
P.O. Box 151439
San Rafael, CA 94915
(415) 453-9800

Also see Mail-Order section, above; several of the organizations listed carry musical selections for relaxation, labor, and postpartum.

PILLOWS

Pillows for Ease
P.O. Box 402113
Miami, FL 33140
(800) 347-1486

Sells cushions and pillows to massage therapists; has one that accommodates a pregnant woman lying on her front. Also sells a special pillow for nursing mothers.

The Right Start Catalog
Right Start Plaza
5334 Sterling Center Dr.
Westlake Village, CA 91361

Sells a pregnancy pillow with two inflatable air chambers that create a hollow area for a pregnant woman's belly.

POSITIONS FOR BIRTH

"Birth Companion," a 16-page pamphlet with pictures of women and their partners in different positions for labor and delivery, and with illustrations of relaxation and massage techniques, is available from Childbirth Graphics Ltd. (see Mail-Order section, above).

POSTPARTUM CARE

National Association of
    Postpartum Care Services
P.O. Box 707
Pittsford, NY 14534

Send SASE.

TENS

American Physical Therapy
    Association
1111 N. Fairfax St.
Alexandria, VA 22314-1488
(703) 684-2782

WATER BIRTH

Book, *Waterbirth: A Gentle Beginning,* available from Birth and Life Bookstore (see Mail-Order section, above), or from:
Gentle Beginnings
P.O Box 1113
Makawao, Maui, HI 96768

Includes instructions on building a birthing tub.

Water Birth International
Barbara Harper
P.O. Box 5554
Santa Barbara, CA 93150
(805) 565-3980

Provides information on water birth. Also rents and sells portable birthing tubs.

References

CHAPTER 1: LABOR PAIN

Bresler, David. *Free Yourself From Pain.* New York: Simon and Schuster, 1979.

Brown, Sylvia T., et al. "Characteristics of Labor Pain at Two Stages of Cervical Dilatation," *Pain* 38(1989):289.

Browning, A.J.F., et al. "Maternal Plasma Concentrations of Beta-Lipotrophin, Beta-Endorphin and Gamma-Lipotrophin Throughout Pregnancy," *British Journal of Obstetrics and Gynaecology* 90(1983):1147.

Cartwright, Ann. "Mothers' Experiences of Induction," *British Medical Journal* 2(1977):745.

Cogan, Rosemary. "Backache in Prepared Childbirth," *Birth and the Family Journal* 3:2(1976):75.

Cogan, Rosemary, and Joseph A. Spinnato. "Pain and Discomfort Thresholds in Late Pregnancy," *Pain* 27(1986):63.

Crowe, Kathryn, and Carl von Baeyer. "Predictors of a Positive Childbirth Experience," *Birth* 16:2(1989):59.

Davis, Joel. *Endorphins.* Garden City, New York: Doubleday, 1984.

"Endorphins and Analgesia," *ICEA Review* 4:3(1980).

Facchinetti, F., et al. "Fetomaternal Opioid Levels and Parturition," *Obstetrics and Gynecology* 62:6(1983):765.

Fox, Howard A. "The Effects of Catecholamine and Drug Treatment on the Fetus and Newborn," *Birth and the Family Journal* 6:3(1979):157.

Gaston-Johansson, Fannie, et al. "Progression of Labor Pain in Primiparas and Multiparas," *Nursing Research* 37:2(1988):86.

Herbert, W. "Placebo: Killing Pain without Opiates," *Science News* 124(Dec. 3, 1983):359.

Kitzinger, Sheila. *The Complete Book of Pregnancy and Childbirth*, revised edition. New York: Alfred A. Knopf, 1989.

Kofinas, George D., et al. "Maternal and Fetal Beta-Endorphin Release in Response to the Stress of Labor and Delivery," *American Journal of Obstetrics and Gynecology* 152(1985):56.

Lederman, R.P., et al. "The Relationship of Maternal Anxiety, Plasma Catecholamines, and Plasma Cortisol to Progress in Labor," *American Journal of Obstetrics and Gynecology* 132(1978):495.

Levinson, Gershon, and Sol M. Shnider. "Catecholamines: The Effects of Maternal Fear and its Treatment on Uterine Function and Circulation," *Birth and the Family Journal* 6:3(1979):167.

Melzack, Ronald, and Eliane Belanger. "Labor Pain: Correlations with Menstrual Pain and Acute Low-Back Pain Before and During Pregnancy," *Pain* 36(1989):225.

Melzack, Ronald, and David Schaffelberg. "Low-Back Pain During Labor," *American Journal of Obstetrics and Gynecology* 156(1987):901.

Melzack, Ronald, and Patrick D. Wall. *The Challenge of Pain.* New York: Basic Books, 1983.

Melzack, Ronald, et al. "Labour is Still Painful after Prepared Childbirth Training," *Canadian Medical Association Journal* 124:5(1981):357.

Melzack, Ronald, et al. "Severity of Labour Pain: Influence of Physical as well as Psychological Variables," *Canadian Medical Association Journal* 130:5(1984):579.

Morgan, William P. "The Mind of the Marathoner," *Psychology Today* (Apr. 1978):39.

Niven, C., and K. Gysbers. "A Study of Labour Pain Using the McGill Pain Questionnaire," *Social Science and Medicine* 19(1984):1347.

Norr, Kathleen, et al. "The Second Time Around: Parity and Birth Experience," *JOGN Nursing* 9(Jan. 1980):30.

Senden, I.P.M. "Labor Pain: A Comparison of Parturients in a Dutch and an American Teaching Hospital," *Obstetrics and Gynecology* 71(1988):541.

Smith, Adam. "The Euphoria of the Long-Distance Swimmer," *Psychology Today* (Apr. 1976):48.

Spanos, Nicholas P., et al. "Hypnosis, Suggestion, and Placebo in the Reduction of Experimental Pain," *Journal of Abnormal Psychology* 98(1989):285.

Suinn, Richard. "Body Thinking: Psychology for Olympic Champs," *Psychology Today* (Jul. 1976):38.

Sundin, Julia. "The Presence of Pain," *International Journal of Childbirth Education* 3:3(1988):16.

Yarrow, Leah. "When My Baby Was Born," *Parents* (Aug. 1982):43.

CHAPTER 2: THE MYTH OF THE PAINLESS BIRTH

Arms, Suzanne. *Immaculate Deception.* Boston: Houghton Mifflin, 1975.

Barrett, Nina. *I Wish Someone Had Told Me.* New York: Simon and Schuster, 1990.

Bresler, David. *Free Yourself from Pain.* New York: Simon and Schuster, 1979.

Dick-Read, Grantly. *Childbirth without Fear.* New York: Harper and Brothers, 1944.

Inch, Sally. *Birthrights.* New York: Random House, 1984.

Jordan, Brigitte. *Birth in Four Cultures.* Montreal: Eden Press, 1983.

Karmel, Marjorie. *Thank You, Dr. Lamaze.* Philadelphia: J.B. Lippincott, 1959.

Lamaze, Fernand. *Painless Childbirth.* New York: Pocket Books, 1965.

Macfarlane, Aidan. *The Psychology of Childbirth.* Cambridge: Harvard University Press, 1977.

McCaffery, Margo. *Nursing Management of the Patient with Pain,* second edition. Philadelphia: J.B. Lippincott, 1979.

Mead, Margaret, and Niles Newton. "Cultural Patterning of Perinatal Behavior," in *Childrearing: Its Social and Psychological Aspects,* S.A. Richardson and A.F. Guttmacher, eds. Baltimore: Williams and Wilkins, 1967.

Morgan, Barbara. "Analgesia and Satisfaction in Childbirth," *Lancet II* 8302(Oct. 9, 1982):808.

Sandelowski, Margarete. *Pain, Pleasure and American Childbirth.* Westport, Conn.: Greenwood, 1984.

Tanzer, Deborah. *Why Natural Childbirth?* Garden City, New York: Doubleday, 1972.

CHAPTER 3: CHILDBIRTH EDUCATION:
The More You Know, The Less It Hurts

Baby Products Tracking Study, 1990, cited in "American Baby Basket," *Parent Trends,* July/August 1991.

Balaskas, Janet. *Active Birth.* Boston: Harvard Common Press, 1992.

Barnes, Fran, and Patricia Hassid. "Bradley/Lamaze," *Childbirth Educator* 5(Fall 1985):40.

Battaglin, Jean. "Lamaze Childbirth: More Than Breathing Lessons," *Genesis* 6(Dec. 1984):23.

Bean, Constance. *Methods of Childbirth,* revised edition. New York: Morrow, 1990.

Bernardini, Judith Y., et al. "Neuromuscular Control of Childbirth: Prepared Women During the First Stage of Labor," *JOGN Nursing* 12(Mar. 1983):105.

Bing, Elisabeth. *Six Practical Lessons for an Easier Childbirth.* New York: Grosset and Dunlap, 1967.

Bradley, Robert. *Husband-Coached Childbirth,* third edition. New York: Harper and Row, 1981.

Brewer, Gail Sforza. *Nine Months, Nine Lessons.* New York: Simon and Schuster, 1983.

Cogan, Rosemary. "Practice Time in Prepared Childbirth," *JOGN Nursing* 7(Jan. 1978):33.

Crowe, Kathryn and Carl von Baeyer. "Predictors of a Positive Childbirth Experience," *Birth* 16:2(1989):59.

Edwards, Margot, and Mary Waldorf. *Reclaiming Birth.* Trumansburg, New York: The Crossing Press, 1984.

Egbert, L.D., et al. "Reduction of Postoperative Pain by Encouragement and Instruction of Patients," *New England Journal of Medicine* 270(1964): 825.

Gamper, Margaret. *Preparation for the Heir Minded,* revised edition. Hammond, Indiana: Sheffield Press, 1973.

Genest, Myles. "Preparation for Childbirth—Evidence for Efficacy: A Review," *JOGN Nursing* 10(Mar. 1981):82.

Gennaro, Susan. "The Childbirth Experience," in *Childbirth Education: Practice, Research, and Theory,* F.H. Nichols and S.S. Humenick, eds. Philadelphia: W.B. Saunders, 1988.

Hetherington, S.E. "A Controlled Study of the Effect of Prepared Childbirth Classes on Obstetric Outcomes," *Birth* 17:2(1990):86.

Humenick, Sharron. "Teaching Relaxation," *Childbirth Educator* 3(Summer 1984):47.

Jiminez, Sherry L.M., "Supportive Pain Management Strategies," in *Childbirth Education: Practice, Research, and Theory,* F.H. Nichols and S.S. Humenick, eds. Philadelphia: W.B. Saunders, 1988.

Kitzinger, Sheila. The Complete Book of Pregnancy and Childbirth, revised edition. New York: Alfred A. Knopf, 1989.

McCaffery, Margo. *Nursing Management of the Patient with Pain,* second edition. Philadelphia: J.B. Lippincott, 1979.

McCutcheon-Rosegg, Susan, and Peter Rosegg. *Natural Childbirth, The Bradley Way.* New York: E.P. Dutton, 1984.

Noble, Elizabeth. *Childbirth with Insight.* Boston: Houghton Mifflin, 1983.

Noble, Elizabeth. *Essential Exercises for the Childbearing Year,* third edition. Boston: Houghton Mifflin, 1988.

Odent, Michel. *Birth Reborn.* New York: Pantheon, 1984.

Odent, Michel. *Water and Sexuality.* London: Penguin, 1990.

Panuthos, Claudia. *Transformation Through Birth.* South Hadley, Massachusetts: Bergin and Garvey, 1984.

Perez, Paulina. "The Importance of Choosing a Qualified Childbirth Educator," *Genesis* 5(Aug. 1983):20.

Peterson, Gayle. *Birthing Normally,* second edition. Berkeley: Mindbody Press, 1984.

Stevens, Richard J. "Psychological Strategies for Management of Pain in Prepared Childbirth, I and II," *Birth and the Family Journal* 3:4(Winter 1976):157, and 4:1(Spring 1977):4.

"Survey of Obstetric and Newborn Services—1989." American Hospital Association, 840 N. Lake Shore Drive, Chicago, Illinois 60611.

Tanzer, Deborah. "Natural Childbirth: Pain or Peak Experience," *Psychology Today* (Oct. 1978):18.

Wideman, Margaret V., and Jerome E. Singer. "The Role of Psychological Mechanisms in Preparation for Childbirth," *American Psychologist* 39(Dec. 1984):1357.

Worthington, Everett L. "Which Prepared-Childbirth Coping Strategies Are Effective?" *JOGN Nursing* 11(Jan. 1982):45.

Yarrow, Leah. "Meet Dr. Bradley," *Parents* (Mar. 1982):61.

CHAPTER 4: LETTING LABOR HAPPEN: Relaxation

Benson, Herbert. *The Relaxation Response.* New York: Morrow, 1975.

Bresler, David. *Free Yourself From Pain.* New York: Simon and Schuster, 1979.

Gamper, Margaret. *Preparation for the Heir Minded,* revised edition. Hammond, Indiana: Sheffield Press, 1973.

Hafen, Brent Q., and Kathryn J. Frandsen. "Autogenic Training," in *From Acupuncture to Yoga: Alternative Methods of Healing.* Englewood Cliffs, New Jersey: Prentice-Hall, 1983.

Humenick, Sharron. "Teaching Relaxation," *Childbirth Educator* 3(Summer 1984):47.

Jacobson, Edmund. *How to Relax and Have Your Baby.* New York: McGraw-Hill, 1959.

Jacobson, Edmund. *You Must Relax,* fourth edition. New York: McGraw-Hill, 1957.

Kitzinger, Sheila. *The Complete Book of Pregnancy and Childbirth,* revised edition. New York: Alfred A. Knopf, 1989.

Kitzinger, Sheila. *The Experience of Childbirth,* fifth edition. New York: Viking Penguin, 1984.

Libresco, Marilyn Maillet. "Relaxation: Progressive and Selective Relaxation," in *Childbirth Education: Practice, Research, and Theory,* F.H. Nichols and S.S. Humenick, eds. Philadelphia: W.B. Saunders, 1988.
McCaffery, Margo. *Nursing Management of the Patient with Pain,* second edition. Philadelphia: J.B. Lippincott, 1979.
Mitchell, Laura. *Simple Relaxation.* London: Murray, 1989.
"Relaxation," *ICEA Sharing* 10(May 1983).

CHAPTER 5: GENTLE INSPIRATION: Breathing For Labor

Barnes, Fran, and Patricia Hassid. "Bradley/Lamaze," *Childbirth Educator* 5(Fall 1985):40.
Caldeyro-Barcia, Roberto. "The Influence of Maternal Bearing-Down Efforts During Second Stage on Fetal Well-Being," *Birth and the Family Journal* 6:1(1979):17.
Grossman, Paul. "Respiration, Stress and Cardiovascular Function," *Psychophysiology* 20(1983):284.
Harris, Victor, et al. "Paced Respiration as a Technique for the Modification of Autonomic Response to Stress," *Psychophysiology* 13(1976):386.
Hilbers, Suzanna May. "Paced Breathing: Terminology Changes and Teaching Techniques," *Genesis* 5(Dec. 1983):16.
Kitzinger, Sheila. *The Complete Book of Pregnancy and Childbirth,* revised edition. New York: Alfred A. Knopf, 1989.
Lane, J.D. "The Effect of Self-Control of Respiration upon Experimental Pain," *Psychophysiology* 18(1981):162.
Mahan, Charles S., and Susan McKay. "Are We Overmanaging Second-Stage Labor?" *Contemporary Ob/Gyn*(Dec. 1984):37.
Noble, Elizabeth. *Essential Exercises for the Childbearing Year,* third edition. Boston: Houghton Mifflin, 1988.
Olkin, Sylvia Klein. *Positive Pregnancy Through Yoga.* Englewood Cliffs, New Jersey: Prentice-Hall, 1981.
Roberts, Joyce, E., et al. "A Descriptive Analysis of Involuntary Bearing-Down Efforts During the Expulsive Phase of Labor," *Journal of Obstetric, Gynecologic and Neonatal Nursing* 16(1987):48.
Rose, Anne Tucker, and Suzanna M. Hilbers. "Relaxation: Paced Breathing Techniques," in *Childbirth Education: Practice, Research, and Theory,* F.H. Nichols and S.S. Humenick, eds. Philadelphia: W.B. Saunders, 1988.

INTRODUCTION TO CHAPTERS 6 – 16

Niven, C., and K. Gysbers. "A Study of Labour Pain Using the McGill Pain Questionnaire," *Social Science and Medicine* 19(1984):1347.

CHAPTER 6: YOU ARE WHAT YOU EAT:
Nutrition Before and After Labor

Broach, Jeannine, and Niles Newton. "Food and Beverages in Labor. Part I: Cross-Cultural and Historical Practices," *Birth* 15:2(1988):81.
Chima, Cinda S. "Healthy Choices for Two," *Lamaze Parents Magazine* (1991):26.

Davis, Adelle. *Let's Have Healthy Children.* New York: New American Library, 1972.

Frame, W.T., et al. "Effect of Nalaxone on Gastric Emptying during Labor," *British Journal of Anaesthesia* 56(1984):263.

Goldbeck, Nikki. "As You Eat, So Your Baby Grows." Ceres Press, Box 87, Dept. D, Woodstock, N.Y. 12498.

Hazle, Nancy R. "Hydration in Labor," *Journal of Nurse-Midwifery* 31(Jul. 1986):171.

Jordan, Brigitte. *Birth in Four Cultures.* Montreal: Eden Press, 1983.

Kaplan, Michael, et al. "Fasting and the Precipitation of Labor: The Yom Kippur Effect," *Journal of the American Medical Association* 250(1983): 1317.

Letters to the Editor, *Mothering,* Fall, 1984.

McKay, Susan, and Charles Mahan. "How Can Aspiration of Vomitus in Obstetrics Best Be Prevented?" *Birth* 15:4(1988):222.

McKay, Susan, and Charles Mahan. "Modifying the Stomach Contents of Laboring Women: Why and How; Success and Risks," *Birth* 15:4(1988): 213.

Marx, Gertie F. "Prevention and Treatment of Aspiration of Gastric Contents," in *The Anesthesiologist, Mother, and Newborn,* S.M. Shnider and F. Moya, eds. Baltimore: Williams and Wilkins, 1974.

Mead, Margaret, and Niles Newton. "Cultural Patterning of Perinatal Behavior," in *Childbearing: Its Social and Psychological Aspects,* S.A. Richardson and A.F. Guttmacher, eds. Baltimore: Williams and Wilkins, 1967.

Simkin, Penny, et al. *Pregnancy, Childbirth, and the Newborn: The Complete Guide,* revised edition. Deephaven, Minn.: Meadowbrook Press, 1991.

Chapter 7: GETTING A BUZZ ON: TENS and Acupuncture

TENS

Augustinsson, Lars-Erik, et al. "Pain Relief During Delivery by Transcutaneous Electrical Nerve Stimulation," *Pain* 4(1977):59.

Dougherty, Ronald J. "TENS: An Alternative to Drugs in the Treatment of Chronic Pain," Paper presented at the General Scientific Meeting, American Pain Society, September, 1979, San Diego, California.

Dunn, P.A., et al. "Transcutaneous Electrical Nerve Stimulation at Acupuncture Points in the Induction of Uterine Contractions," *Obstetrics and Gynecology* 73(1989):286.

Grim, Louise C. and Susan H. Morey. "Transcutaneous Electrical Nerve Stimulation for Relief of Parturition Pain: A Clinical Report," *Physical Therapy* 65(Mar. 1985):337.

Harrison, Robert F., et al. "Pain Relief in Labour Using TENS," *British Journal of Obstetrics and Gynecology* 93(1986):739.

Keenan, Donna, et al. "Transcutaneous Electrical Nerve Stimulation for Pain Control During Labor and Delivery: A Case Report," *Physical Therapy* 65(Sept. 1985):1363.

Mannheimer, Jeffrey S. and Gerald N. Lampe. *Clinical Transcutaneous Electrical Nerve Stimulation.* Philadelphia: F.A. Davis, 1984.

Moore, Debra Eitelman, and H. Martin Blacker. "How Effective is TENS for Chronic Pain?" *American Journal of Nursing* 83(Aug. 1983):1175.

Robson, J.E. "Transcutaneous Nerve Stimulation for Pain Relief in Labour," *Anaesthesia* 34(1979):357.

Stewart, P. "Transcutaneous Nerve Stimulation as a Method of Analgesia in Labour," *Anaesthesia* 34(1979):361.

"TENS in Pregnancy, Labor and Delivery." Special Issue, *Journal of Obstetric and Gynecologic Physical Therapy* 12:3(Sept. 1988).

Acupuncture

"Acupuncture: A Curious Cure that Works," *Changing Times* (Nov. 1980):37.

Editorial, "How Does Acupuncture Work?" *British Medical Journal* 283(Sept. 19, 1981):746.

Hassett, James. "Acupuncture is Proving its Points," *Psychology Today* (Dec. 1980):81.

Ho, Mobi. "Acupuncture in Pregnancy," *Mothering* (Summer 1984):61.

Kotzsch, Ronald E. "Acupuncture Today," *East West Journal* 16(Jan. 1986): 58.

National Symposia of Acupuncture and Moxibustion and Acupuncture Anesthesia, Beijing, Jun. 1979.

Wallis, Claudia. "Why New Age Medicine is Catching On," *Time* 138:18 (Nov. 4, 1991):68.

CHAPTER 8: RUBBING WHERE IT HURTS:
Massage, Counterpressure, and Acupressure

Avery, Melissa, and B.A. Burket. "Effect of Perineal Massage on the Incidence of Episiotomy and Perineal Laceration in a Nurse Midwifery Service," *Journal of Nurse-Midwifery* 31(1986):128.

Avery, Melissa, and Laura Van Arsdale. "Perineal Massage," *Journal of Nurse-Midwifery* 32(1987):181.

Balaskas, Janet. *Natural Pregnancy.* New York: Interlink, 1990.

Chan, Pedro. *Finger Acupressure.* New York: Random House, 1985.

Cain, Kathy. *Partners in Birth.* New York: Warner, 1990.

Flaws, Bob. *The Path of Pregnancy.* Boulder, Colo.: Blue Poppy Press, 1982.

Inkeles, Gordon. *Massage and Peaceful Pregnancy.* New York: Putnam, 1984.

Jiminez, Sherry L.M. "Acupressure: Hands-On Pain Relief," *Genesis* (Jun./Jul. 1990):4.

Jiminez, Sherry L.M. "Beating the Pain of Childbirth," *American Baby* (May 1991):36.

Jiminez, Sherry L.M. "Relaxation: Acupressure," in *Childbirth Education: Practice, Research, and Theory,* F.H. Nichols and S.S. Humenick, eds. Philadelphia: W.B. Saunders, 1988.

Montagu, Ashley. *Touching,* second edition. New York: Harper and Row, 1978.

Moss, Suzan. "The Ancient Art of Applying Pressure Where it Counts," *Dance Magazine* (May 1982):143.

Ohashi, Wataru, with Mary Hoover. *Natural Childbirth, the Eastern Way.* New York: Ballantine, 1983.

Rosenbaum, Ron. "Shiatsu: The Pressure is On," *Esquire* (Sept. 1984):304.

Simkin, Penny. *The Birth Partner.* Boston: Harvard Common Press, 1989.

Simkin, Penny. "Prenatal Perineal Massage," Appendix A in *Episiotomy and the Second Stage of Labor,* second edition, Sheila Kitzinger and Penny Simkin, eds. Seattle: Pennypress, 1986.
Sorel, Nancy. *Ever Since Eve.* New York: Oxford University Press, 1984.
Stern, Zelda. "Shiatsu," *Childbirth Educator* 1(Summer 1982):20.

CHAPTER 9: SOME LIKE IT HOT, SOME LIKE IT COLD: Water

Ader, Lena, et al. "Parturition Pain Treated by Intracutaneous Injections of Sterile Water," *Pain* 41(1990):133.
Bresler, David. *Free Yourself from Pain.* New York: Simon and Schuster, 1979.
Church, Linda K. "Water Birth: One Birthing Center's Observations," *Journal of Nurse-Midwifery* 34(1989):165.
Clark, Matt. "Giving Birth Under Water," *Newsweek* (Jan. 16, 1984):70.
Lenstrup, C., et al. "Warm Tub Baths During Delivery," *Acta Obstetrica et Gynecologica Scandinavica* 66(1987):709.
McCaffery, Margo. *Nursing Management of the Patient with Pain,* revised edition. Philadelphia: J.B. Lippincott, 1979.
Melzack, Ronald, and Patrick D. Wall. *The Challenge of Pain.* New York: Basic Books, 1983.
Melzack, Ronald, et al. "Relief of Dental Pain by Ice Massage of the Hand," *Canadian Medical Association Journal* 122(Jan. 26, 1980):189.
Odent, Michel. *Birth Reborn.* New York: Pantheon, 1984.
Odent, Michel. "Birth Under Water," *Lancet* II 8365/6(Dec. 24, 1983):1476.
Odent, Michel. "The Evolution of Obstetrics at Pithiviers," *Birth and the Family Journal* 8:1(1981):7.
Odent, Michel. *Water and Sexuality.* New York: Penguin, 1990.
Ray, Sondra. *Ideal Birth,* revised edition. Berkeley: Celestial Arts, 1987.
Rivers, Anne. *Waterbirth: A Gentle Beginning* (1988). Gentle Beginnings, P.O. Box 1113, Makawao, Maui, Hawaii 96768.
Simkin, Penny. "Comfort Measures for Labor and How They Work," *International Journal of Childbirth Education* 2:2(1987):5.
Trolle, B., et al. "The Effect of Sterile Water Blocks on Low Back Labor Pain," *American Journal of Obstetrics and Gynecology* 164(1991):1277.

CHAPTER 10: DON'T TAKE IT LYING DOWN: Activity

Balaskas, Janet. *Active Birth,* revised edition. Boston: Harvard Common Press, 1992.
Biancuzzo, Marie. "The Patient Observer: Does the Hands-and-Knees Posture During Labor Help to Rotate the Occiput Posterior Fetus?" *Birth* 18:1(1991):40.
Carlson, Jerold M., et al. "Maternal Position," *Obstetrics and Gynecology* 68 (1986):443.
Clapp, J.F. III. "The Course of Labor After Endurance Exercise During Pregnancy," *American Journal of Obstetrics and Gynecology* 163(1990):1799.
Dundes, Lauren. "The Evolution of Maternal Birth Position," *American Journal of Public Health* 77(1987):636.
Fenwick, Loel. "Birthing Positions," *Lamaze Parents Magazine* (1991):54.
Kurokawa, Jude, and Mark Zilkoski. "Adapting Hospital Obstetrics to Birth in the Squatting Position," *Birth* 12:2(1985):87.

McKay, Susan, and Joyce Roberts. "Maternal Position During Labor and Birth: What Have We Learned?" *ICEA Review* 13:2(Aug. 1989).

Noble, Elizabeth. *Childbirth with Insight.* Boston: Houghton Mifflin, 1983.

Noble, Elizabeth. *Essential Exercises for the Childbearing Year,* third edition. Boston: Houghton Mifflin, 1988.

Nodine, Priscilla, and Joyce Roberts. "Factors Associated With Perineal Outcome During Childbirth," *Journal of Nurse-Midwifery* 32(May/Jun. 1987):123.

Roberts, Joyce. "Debate: Which Position for the First Stage?" *Childbirth Educator* 1:4(1982):35.

Roberts, Joyce, and Donna van Lier. "Debate: Which Position for the Second Stage?" *Childbirth Educator* 3:3(1984):33.

Simkin, Penny. Letter, *Birth* 9:1(1982):49.

Simkin, Penny, et al. *Pregnancy, Childbirth, and the Newborn,* revised edition. Deephaven, Minn.: Meadowbrook, 1991.

Varassi, Guistino, et al. "Effects of Physical Activity on Maternal Plasma Beta Endorphin Levels and Perception of Labor Pain," *American Journal of Obstetrics and Gynecology* 160(1989):707.

CHAPTER 11: EVERYTHING BUT THE KITCHEN SINK:
Comfort Devices to Bring to the Hospital

Ulrich, Roger S. "View Through a Window May Influence Recovery from Surgery," *Science* 224(Apr. 27, 1984):421.

CHAPTER 12: LISTENING TO YOUR BODY: Biofeedback

Blai, Boris. "Biofeedback: Is it for You?" *Journal of American College Health* 33(1985):217.

Bresler, David. *Free Yourself from Pain.* New York: Simon and Schuster, 1979.

Bridgwater, Carol Austin. "Warm Hands and Children's Migraines," *Psychology Today* (Jan. 1985):71.

Brown, Barbara A. *Stress and the Art of Biofeedback.* New York: Harper and Row, 1977.

Danskin, David A., and Mark A. Crow. *Biofeedback: An Introduction and Guide.* Palo Alto: Mayfield, 1981.

DiFranco, Joyce. "Relaxation: Biofeedback," in *Childbirth Education: Practice, Research, and Theory,* F.H. Nichols and S.S. Humenick, eds. Philadelphia: W.B. Saunders, 1988.

Duchene, Pam. "Using Biofeedback to Ease the Pain of Childbirth," *American Journal of Nursing* 89(Aug. 1989):1070B.

Melzack, Ronald, and Patrick D. Wall. *The Challenge of Pain.* New York: Basic Books, 1983.

Proctor, Mark R., and Carol A. Warfield. "Biofeedback Pain Control," *Hospital Practice* 19(Apr. 1984):104D.

St. James-Roberts, Ian, et al. "Biofeedback as an Aid to Childbirth," *British Journal of Obstetrics and Gynaecology* 90(1983):56.

Warga, Claire. "Little Swamis," *Psychology Today* (Jan. 1985):16.

CHAPTER 13: MIND OVER MATTER:
Visualization, Hypnosis, and Therapeutic Touch

Bates, Brian, and Allison Newman Turner. "Imagery and Symbolism in the Birth Practices of Traditional Cultures," *Birth* 12(Spring 1985):29.

Battaglin, Jean. "Lamaze Childbirth—More than Breathing Lessons," *Genesis* 6(Dec. 1984):23.

Bradley, Robert. *Husband-Coached Childbirth*, third edition. New York: Harper and Row, 1981.

Bresler, David. *Free Yourself from Pain*. New York: Simon and Schuster, 1979.

Brown, Michael. "The Psychic Search," *American Health* (Nov. 1985):64.

Bry, Adelaide. *Directing the Movies of Your Mind*. New York: Harper and Row, 1978.

Copelan, Rachel. *How to Hypnotize Yourself and Others*. New York: Harper and Row, 1982.

Cousins, Norman. *Anatomy of an Illness*. New York: Norton, 1979.

DiFranco, Joyce. "The Use of Guided Imagery in Preterm Labor," in *Expanding Horizons in Childbirth Education*, Donna Ewy, ed. Arlington, Virginia: ASPO/Lamaze, 1985.

Fanning, Patrick. *Visualization for Change*. Oakland, Calif.: New Harbinger Publications, 1988.

Freeman, R.M., et al. "Randomised Trial of Self-Hypnosis for Analgesia in Labour," *British Medical Journal* 292(Mar. 8, 1986):657.

Garfield, Patricia. *Creative Dreaming*. New York: Ballantine, 1985.

Harcus, Sue. "Baby's Birth Medical First," *The Journal Times,* Racine, Wisconsin (Oct. 15, 1978):1E.

Hilgard, Ernest R. "A Study in Hypnosis," *Psychology Today* (Jan. 1986):23.

Hilgard, Ernest R., and Josephine R. Hilgard. *Hypnosis in the Relief of Pain*. Los Altos, Calif.: William Kaufmann, 1975.

Hook, Lynne O'Neill. *Hypnotizing Yourself for Success* (1988). R&E Publishers, P.O. Box 2008, Saratoga, CA 95070.

Jones, Carl. *Mind Over Labor*. New York: Viking Penguin, 1987.

Jones, Carl. *Visualizations for an Easier Childbirth*. Deephaven, Minn.: Meadowbrook Press, 1988.

Kitzinger, Sheila. *Women as Mothers*. New York: Vintage, 1980.

Knaster, Mirka. "Dolores Krieger's Therapeutic Touch," *East/West* (Aug. 1989):54.

Krieger, Dolores. *Therapeutic Touch*. Englewood Cliffs, New Jersey: Prentice-Hall, 1979.

Lawson, Carol. "Sick Children Learn Self-Hypnotism to Fight Pain," *New York Times* (Sept. 8, 1985).

Levine, Stephen. *Who Dies?* New York: Doubleday, 1982.

Lothian, Judith. "Relaxation: Therapeutic Touch," in *Childbirth Education: Practice, Research, and Theory*, F.H. Nichols and S.S. Humenick, eds. Philadelphia: W.B. Saunders, 1988.

McCaffery, Margo. *Nursing Management of the Patient with Pain*, second edition. Philadelphia: J.B. Lippincott, 1979.

Maybruck, Patricia. *Pregnancy and Dreams*. Los Angeles: Jeremy P. Tarcher, 1989.

Melzack, Ronald, and Patrick D. Wall. *The Challenge of Pain*. New York: Basic Books, 1983.

Olness, Karen. "Hypnotherapy: A Cyberphysiologic Strategy in Pain Management," in *Acute Pain in Children (Pediatric Clinics of North America* 36), N.L. Schechter, ed., 1989.

Peterson, Gayle. *Birthing Normally,* second edition. Berkeley: Mindbody Press, 1984.

Samuels, Mike, and Nancy Samuels. *Seeing with the Mind's Eye.* New York: Random House, 1975.

Silva, Jose. *The Silva Mind Control Method.* New York: Pocket Books, 1989.

Simonton, O. Carl, et al. *Getting Well Again.* New York: Bantam, 1982.

Smoller, Bruce, and Brian Schulman. *Pain Control: The Bethesda Program.* Garden City, New York: Doubleday, 1982.

Spanos, Nicholas P., et al. "Hypnosis, Suggestion, and Placebo in the Reduction of Experimental Pain," *Journal of Abnormal Psychology* 98(1989):285.

Steffes, Sandra. "Imagery: Solving the Mysteries of Appropriate Application," in *Expanding Horizons in Childbirth Education,* Donna Ewy, ed. Arlington, Virginia: ASPO/Lamaze, 1985.

Stern, Zelda. "The Healing Touch," *Childbirth Educator* (Summer 1985):43.

Vadurro, Judith F., and Priscilla A. Butts. "Reducing the Anxiety and Pain of Childbirth through Hypnosis," *American Journal of Nursing* 82(Apr. 1982):620.

Wain, Harold J. "Pain Control Through Use of Hypnosis," *American Journal of Clinical Hypnosis* 23(1980):41.

Wallis, Claudia. "Why New Age Medicine is Catching On," *Time* 138:180 (Nov. 4, 1991):68.

Williams, Wendy. *The Power Within.* New York: Harper and Row, 1990.

Wuitchik, Michael, et al. "The Clinical Significance of Pain and Cognitive Activity in Latent Labor," *Obstetrics and Gynecology* 73(1989):35.

CHAPTER 14: CHARMS TO SOOTHE: Music

Clark, M., et al. "Music Therapy-Assisted Labor and Delivery," *Journal of Music Therapy* 18(1981):88.

DiFranco, Joyce. "Relaxation: Music," in *Childbirth Education: Practice, Research, and Theory,* F.H. Nichols and S.S. Humenick, eds. Philadelphia: W.B. Saunders, 1988.

Gentry, Cheryl. "Use of Music in Childbirth Class," ICEA Teaching Ideas Sheet, *International Journal of Childbirth Education* 5:2(May 1990):32.

Hanser, Suzanne B., et al. "The Effect of Music on the Relaxation of Expectant Mothers During Labor," *Journal of Music Therapy* 20(1983):50.

Kershner, Jody, and Virginia Schenk. "Music Therapy-Assisted Childbirth," *International Journal of Childbirth Education* 6:3(1991):32.

Livingston, Janice C. "Music for the Childbearing Family," *Journal of Obstetric, Gynecologic and Neonatal Nursing* 8(Nov.–Dec. 1979):363.

McCaffery, Margo. *Nursing Management of the Patient with Pain,* second edition. Philadelphia: J.B. Lippincott, 1979.

Melzack, Ronald, and Patrick D. Wall. *The Challenge of Pain.* New York: Basic Books, 1983.

Smith, Richard. "Music to Labour To," *British Medical Journal* 287 (1983): 1984.

Trotter, Robert. "Maybe It's the Music," *Psychology Today* (May 1984):8.

CHAPTER 15: YOU NEED A FRIEND: Companionship

Bertsch, T.D. "Labor Support by First-Time Fathers: Direct Observations," *Journal of Psychosomatic Obstetrics and Gynecology* 11(1990):251.

Block, Carolyn R., and Richard Block. "The Effect of Support of the Husband and Obstetrician on Pain Perception and Control in Childbirth," *Birth and the Family Journal* 2:2(1975):43.

Cain, Kathy. *Partners in Birth*. New York: Warner, 1990.

Campbell, Anne, and Everett L. Worthington. "Teaching Expectant Fathers How to Be Better Childbirth Coaches," *American Journal of Maternal-Child Nursing* 7(Jan.–Feb. 1982):28.

Cogan, Rosemary, et al. "Predictors of Pain During Prepared Childbirth," *Journal of Psychosomatic Research* 20(1976):23.

Cohen, Nancy Wainer, and Lois J. Estner. *Silent Knife*. South Hadley, Mass.: Bergin and Garvey, 1983.

Ettner, Randi. "The Work of Worrying: Emotional Preparation for Labor," in *Pregnancy as Healing*, volume II, G.H. Peterson and Lewis Mehl, eds. Berkeley: Mindbody Press, 1985.

Gaskin, Ina May. *Spiritual Midwifery*, third edition. Summertown, Tenn.: The Book Publishing Company, 1990.

"Harper's Index," *Harper's* (Aug. 1985).

Henneborn, W.J., and Rosemary Cogan. "The Effect of Husband Participation on Reported Pain and Probability of Medication During Labor and Birth," *Journal of Psychosomatic Research* 19(1975):215.

Hotelling, Barbara A. "Labor Support/Doulas: Questions and Answers," *ICEA Forum/Sharing* 1:2(1985):13.

Hotelling, Barbara A. "Labor Support Makes it a Labor of Love," *ICEA Forum/Sharing* 1:1(1985):15.

Jones, Carl. *Sharing Birth*. South Hadley, Mass.: Bergin and Garvey, 1989.

Jordan, Brigitte. *Birth in Four Cultures*. Montreal: Eden Press, 1983.

Kennell, John H., et al. "Continuous Emotional Support During Labor in a U.S. Hospital: A Randomized Controlled Trial," *Journal of the American Medical Association* 265(1991):2197.

Kennell, John H. "The Physiologic Effects of a Supportive Companion (Doula) During Labor," in *Birth, Interaction and Attachment*, M.H. Klaus and M.O. Robertson, eds. Skillman, New Jersey: Johnson and Johnson, 1982.

Klaus, Marshall H., and Kennell, John H. *Parent-Infant Bonding*, second edition. St. Louis: C.V. Mosby, 1982.

Klein, Robert P., et al. "A Study of Father and Nurse Support During Labor," *Birth and the Family Journal* 8:3(1981):161.

Korte, Diana, and Roberta Scaer. *A Good Birth, A Safe Birth,* revised edition. Boston: Harvard Common Press, 1992.

Lozoff, Betsy. "Birth in Non-Industrial Societies," in *Birth, Interaction and Attachment*, M.H. Klaus and M.O. Robertson, eds. Skillman, New Jersey: Johnson and Johnson, 1982.

Lucey, Marilyn. "Why Hire Labor Support?" *C/SEC Newsletter* 11:2 (1985):1.

Mosedale, Laura. "Fathers in the Delivery Room," *Self* (April 1991):104.

Peddicord, Karen, et al. "An Independent Labor-Support Nursing Service," *Journal of Obstetric, Gynecologic and Neonatal Nursing* 13(Sept. 1984):312.

Perez, Paulina and Cheryl Snedeker. *Special Women: The Role of the Professional Labor Assistant.* Seattle: Pennypress, 1990.

Peterson, Gayle H., and Lewis Mehl. *Pregnancy as Healing,* volume II. Berkeley: Mindbody Press, 1985.

Raphael, Dana. *The Tender Gift: Breastfeeding.* New York: Schocken, 1976.

Shearer, Beth. "Birth Assistant: New Ally for Parents-to-Be," *Childbirth Educator* 8:3(1989):26.

Simkin, Penny. *The Birth Partner.* Boston: Harvard Common Press, 1989.

Sosa, Roberto, et al. "The Effect of a Supportive Companion on Perinatal Problems, Length of Labor, and Mother-Infant Interaction," *New England Journal of Medicine* 303(1980):597.

Stephany, Theresa. "Supporting the Mother of a Patient in Labor," *Journal of Obstetric, Gynecologic and Neonatal Nursing* 12(1983):345.

"Support During Labor: Good Common Sense," *ICEA Review* (Apr. 1984).

"Survey of Obstetric and Newborn Services—1989," American Hospital Association, 840 N. Lake Shore Drive, Chicago, Ill. 60611.

Tanzer, Deborah. *Why Natural Childbirth?* Garden City, New York: Doubleday, 1972.

Van der Meer, Antonia. "Doulas: In Service Of...," *Childbirth Instructor* 1:3(1991):28.

Yarrow, Leah. "Fathers Speak Out," *Parents* (Sept. 1985):91.

CHAPTER 16: SETTING THE MOOD: The Birth Environment

Dick-Read, Grantly. *Childbirth Without Fear.* New York: Harper and Brothers, 1944.

Gordon, Suzanne. "My Search for the Perfect Birth," *Mother Jones* (Oct. 1985):32.

Haire, Doris B., and Charlotte Cram Elsberry. "Maternity Care and Outcomes in a High-Risk Service: The North Central Bronx Experience," *Birth* 18:1(1991):33.

Korte, Diana, and Roberta Scaer. *A Good Birth, A Safe Birth,* revised edition. Boston: Harvard Common Press, 1992.

Lesko, Wendy, and Matthew Lesko. *The Maternity Sourcebook.* New York: Warner, 1984.

Mason, Diane. "Options in Hospital Births," *American Baby* (Mar. 1986):49.

Mehl, Lewis. "Research on Alternatives in Childbirth," in *21st Century Obstetrics Now!* volume I, D. Stewart and L. Stewart, eds. Marble Hill, Missouri, 1977.

Newton, Niles, et al. "Effect of Disturbance on Labor," *American Journal of Obstetrics and Gynecology* 101(1968):1096.

Newton, Niles. "Laboring Undisturbed," *Childbirth Educator* 8:2(1988/1989):42.

Odent, Michel. "Introduction," in *Active Birth,* by Janet Balaskas. Boston: Harvard Common Press, 1992.

Odent, Michel. "The Milieu and Obstetrical Positions During Labor: A New Approach from France," in *Birth, Interaction and Attachment,* M.H. Klaus and M.O. Robertson, eds. Skillman, New Jersey: Johnson and Johnson, 1982.

Perry, Phil. "The Obstetrics Market Matures for LDRs/LDRPs," *Health Care Strategic Management* 8:4(1990):1.

Phillips, Celeste. "Single Room Maternity Care for Maximum Cost Efficiency," *Perinatology/Neonatology* 12(Mar.–Apr. 1988):25.

Petty, Roy. *Home Birth.* Northbrook, Illinois: Domus, 1979.

Rooks, Judith. "Outcomes of Care in Birth Centers: The National Birth Center Study," *New England Journal of Medicine* 321(1989):1804.

Schuman, Wendy. "Hospital Birth: How to Get the Best Care," *Parents* (Nov. 1984):204.

CHAPTER 17: HOSPITAL ROUTINES: Is the Gain Worth the Pain?

American College of Obstetricians and Gynecologists, Committee Opinion Number 64, Oct. 1988.

Banta, David, and Stephen B. Thacker. "The Risks and Benefits of Episiotomy," *Birth* 9:1(1982):25.

Berkus, Michael D., et al. "Cohort Study of Silastic Vacuum Cup Deliveries: I. Safety of the Instrument," *Obstetrics and Gynecology* 66(1985):503.

Conway, David I. "Management of Spontaneous Rupture of the Membranes in the Absence of Labor in Primgravid Women at Term," *American Journal of Obstetrics and Gynecology* 150(1984):947.

Dierker, LeRoy J. "The Midforceps: Maternal and Neonatal Outcomes," *American Journal of Obstetrics and Gynecology* 152(1985):176.

Duff, Patrick, et al. "Management of Premature Rupture of the Membranes and Unfavorable Cervix in Term Pregnancy," *Obstetrics and Gynecology* 63(1984):697.

"Electronic Fetal Monitoring, Intermittent Auscultation Found Comparable," *American College of Obstetricians and Gynecologists Newsletter* 32:11(1988):1.

"Episiotomy," *ICEA Review* 9:2(Aug. 1985).

Flamm, Bruce. *Birth After Cesarean.* New York: Prentice-Hall, 1990.

Green, James R., and Sonia L. Soohoo. "Factors Associated with Rectal Injury in Spontaneous Deliveries," *Obstetrics and Gynecology* 73(1989):732.

Harrison, R.F., et al. "Is Routine Episiotomy Necessary?" *British Medical Journal* 288(Jun. 30, 1984):1971.

Hodnett, Ellen. "Patient Control During Labor: Effects of Two Types of Fetal Monitors," *Journal of Obstetric, Gynecologic and Neonatal Nursing* 11(Mar.-Apr. 1982):94.

Johanson, Richard, et al. "North Staffordshire/Wigan Assisted Delivery Trial," *British Journal of Obstetrics and Gynecology* 96(1989):537.

Kitzinger, Sheila, and Penny Simkin. *Episiotomy and the Second Stage of Labor,* revised edition. Seattle: Pennypress, 1986.

Lieberman, Adrienne. "Heads Up: When Your Baby is Breech," *American Baby* (Apr. 1991):80.

Lieberman, Adrienne. "Pitocin: Forced Labor," *American Baby* (May 1990):56.

"Management of Labor Following Rupture of Membranes," *ICEA Review* 8:3 (Dec. 1984).

Mercer, Brian, et al. "Labor Induction with Continuous Low-Dose Oxytocin Infusion: A Randomized Trial," *Obstetrics and Gynecology* 77(1991):659.

Newton, Niles, et al. "Psychological, Physiologic, Nutritional and Technologic Aspects of Intravenous Infusion During Labor," *Birth* 15:2(1988):67.

"Preoperative Depilation," *Lancet I* 8337(Jun. 11, 1983):1311.

Price, Emma. "The Trouble with Fetal Monitoring" (letter), *Parents* (Nov. 1985):12.

Rayburn, William F. "Prostaglandin E2 Gel For Cervical Ripening and Induction of Labor: A Critical Analysis," *American Journal of Obstetrics and Gynecology* 160(1989):529.

Romney, Mona L., and H. Gordon. "Is Your Enema Really Necessary?" *British Medical Journal* 282(Apr. 18, 1981):1269.

Rosen, Mortimer. *The Cesarean Myth.* New York: Penguin, 1989.

Schutte, M.F., et al. "Management of Premature Rupture of Membranes: The Risk of Vaginal Examination to the Infant," *American Journal of Obstetrics and Gynecology* 146(1983):395.

Shiono, Patricia, et al. "Midline Episiotomies—More Harm Than Good?" *Obstetrics and Gynecology* 75(1990):765.

Silver, Lynn, and Sidney M. Wolfe. "Unnecessary Cesarean Sections: How to Cure a National Epidemic," Public Citizens Health Research Group, 2000 P Street NW, Washington, D.C. 20036.

Simkin, Penny. *The Birth Partner.* Boston: Harvard Common Press, 1989.

Simkin, Penny. "Stress, Pain, and Catecholamines in Labor: Part I. A Review, and Part II. Stress Associated with Childbirth Events: A Pilot Study of New Mothers," *Birth* 13:4(1986):234.

Sleep, Jennifer. "West Berkshire Perineal Management Trial," *British Medical Journal* 289(Sept. 8, 1984):587.

Stewart, P. "Spontaneous Labour: When Should the Membranes Be Ruptured?" *British Journal of Obstetrics and Gynaecology* 89(Jan. 1982):39.

Thorp, John M., Jr., and Watson A. Bowes, Jr. "Episiotomy: Can Its Routine Use Be Defended?" *American Journal of Obstetrics and Gynecology* 160(1989):1027.

Thorp, John M., Jr., et al. "Selected Use of Midline Episiotomy: Effect on Perineal Trauma," *Obstetrics and Gynecology* 70(1987):260.

Trofatter, Kenneth F., et al. "Preinduction Cervical Ripening with Prostaglandin E2 (Prepidil) Gel," *American Journal of Obstetrics and Gynecology* 153(1985):268.

Wagner, Michael, et al. "A Comparison of Early and Delayed Induction of Labor with Spontaneous Rupture of Membranes at Term," *Obstetrics and Gynecology* 74(1989):93.

Walker, M.P.R., et al. "Epidural Anesthesia, Episiotomy, and Obstetrical Laceration," *Obstetrics and Gynecology* 77(1991):668.

Wilcox, Lynne S., et al. "Episiotomy and its Role in the Incidence of Perineal Lacerations in a Maternity Center and a Tertiary Hospital Obstetric Service," *American Journal of Obstetrics and Gynecology* 160(1989):1047.

Williams, J. Kell, et al. "Use of Prostaglandin E2 Topical Cervical Gel in High-Risk Patients: A Critical Analysis," *Obstetrics and Gynecology* 66 (1985):769.

Young, Diony, and Charles Mahan. *Unnecessary Cesareans: Ways to Avoid Them,* revised edition. Minneapolis, Minn.: ICEA, 1989.

CHAPTER 18: MEDICAL AIDS

Avard, Denise, and Carl Nimrod. "Risks and Benefits of Obstetric Epidural Analgesia: A Review," *Birth* 12:4(1985):215.

Ericson, Avis J. *Medications Used During Labor and Birth.* Milwaukee, ICEA, 1977.

Fisher, Scott, et al. "Obstetric Analgesia and Anesthesia," in *Management of Labor,* second edition, W.R. Cohen, et al., eds. Rockville, Maryland: Aspen Publishers, 1989.

Fleming, Nancy. "Comparison of Women with Different Perineal Conditions After Childbirth," unpublished doctoral dissertation, University of Illinois at Chicago, 1987.

Fox, Howard A. "The Effects of Catecholamine and Drug Treatment on the Fetus and Newborn," *Birth and the Family Journal* 6:3(1979):157.

Fusi, Luca, et al. "Maternal Pyrexia Associated with the Use of Epidural Analgesia During Labor," *Lancet I*(1989):1250.

Kaminski, H.M., et al. "The Effect of Epidural Analgesia on the Frequency of Instrumental Obstetric Delivery," *Obstetrics and Gynecology* 69(1987):770.

King, Jeffrey, and Donald M. Sherline. "Paracervical and Pudendal Block," *Clinical Obstetrics and Gynecology* 24(Jun. 1981):587.

Kirkpatrick, Sarah, and Russell K. Laros. "Characteristics of Normal Labor," *Obstetrics and Gynecology* 74(1989):85.

Levinson, Gershon, and Sol M. Shnider. "Catecholamines: The Effects of Maternal Fear and Its Treatment on Uterine Function and Circulation," *Birth and the Family Journal* 6:3(1979):167.

Levinson, Gershon, and Sol M. Shnider. "Systemic Medication for Labor and Delivery," in *Anesthesia for Obstetrics,* second edition, S.M. Shnider and G. Levinson, eds. Baltimore: Williams and Wilkins, 1987.

MacArthur, C., et al. "Epidural Anaesthesia and Long-term Backache After Childbirth," *British Medical Journal* 301(1990):9.

Morgan, Barbara M. "Analgesia and Satisfaction in Childbirth," *Lancet II* 8302(Oct. 1982):808.

Murphy, J.D., et al. "Bupivacaine Versus Bupivacaine Plus Fentanyl for Epidural Analgesia—Effect on Maternal Satisfaction," *British Medical Journal* 302(Mar. 9, 1991):564.

Ong, B.Y., et al. "Anesthesia for Cesarean Section—Effects on Neonates," *Anesthesia and Analgesia* 68(1989):270.

Pederson, Hilda, et al. "Obstetric Anesthesia," in *Clinical Anesthesiology,* P.G. Barash et al., eds. Philadelphia: J.B. Lippincott, 1989.

Phillipson, Elliot H., et al. "Maternal, Fetal, and Neonatal Lidocaine Levels Following Local Perineal Infiltration," *American Journal of Obstetrics and Gynecology* 149(1984):403.

Podlas, Jeffrey, and Burnis Breland. "Patient-Controlled Analgesia with Nalbuphine During Labor," *Obstetrics and Gynecology* 70(1987):202.

Shnider, Sol M. "Maternal Catecholamines Decrease During Labor After Lumbar Epidural Anesthesia," *American Journal of Obstetrics and Gynecology* 147(1983):13.

Shnider, Sol M., and Gershon Levinson. "Anesthesia for Cesarean Section," in *Anesthesia for Obstetrics,* second edition, S.M. Shnider and G. Levinson, eds. Baltimore: Williams and Wilkins, 1987.

Thorp, James A., et al. "The Effect of Continuous Epidural Analgesia on Cesarean Section for Dystocia in Nulliparous Women," *American Journal of Obstetrics and Gynecology* 161(1989):670.

Thorp, James A., et al. "Effects of Epidural Analgesia: Some Questions and Answers," *Birth* 17:3(1990):157.

Yarrow, Leah. "When My Baby Was Born," *Parents* 57(Aug. 1982):43.

CHAPTER 19: IS BIRTH PAINFUL FOR THE BABY, TOO?

Blass, Elliott M., and Lisa B. Hoffmeyer. "Sucrose as an Analgesic for Newborn Infants," *Pediatrics* 87(1991):215.

Briggs, Anne. *Circumcision: What Every Parent Should Know* (1985). Birth and Parenting Publications, Rt. 1, Box 137, Earlysville, Virginia 22936.

Brown, M.S. "Circumcision Decision—Prominence of Social Concerns," *Pediatrics* 80(1987):215.

"Circumcision," *ICEA Review* 5:1(Apr. 1981).

Davies, Robertson. *The Rebel Angels*. New York: Viking, 1982.

DeLee, Joseph B. "The Prophylactic Forceps Operation," *American Journal of Obstetrics and Gynecology* 1(1920):32.

Field, Tiffany, and Edward Goldson. "Pacifying Effects of Nonnutritive Sucking on Term and Preterm Neonates During Heelstick Procedures," *Pediatrics* 74(1984):1012.

Gardner, Sherry. "The Mother as Incubator After Delivery," *Journal of Obstetric, Gynecologic and Neonatal Nursing* 8(May–Jun. 1979):174.

Henningson, Annelie, et al. "Bathing or Washing Babies After Birth?" *Lancet* II 8260/1(Dec. 19/26, 1981):1401.

Herrera, Alfredo J. "The Role of Parental Information in the Incidence of Circumcision," *Pediatrics* 70(1982):597.

Holve, Richard L., et al. "Regional Anesthesia During Newborn Circumcision," *Clinical Pediatrics* 22(1983):813.

Hunziker, Urs A., and Ronald G. Barr. "Increased Carrying Reduces Infant Crying: A Randomized Controlled Trial," *Pediatrics* 77(1986):641.

Jones, Sandy. *Crying Baby, Sleepless Nights,* revised edition. Boston: Harvard Common Press, 1992.

Kitzinger, Sheila. *The Complete Book of Pregnancy and Childbirth,* revised edition. New York: Alfred A. Knopf, 1989.

Klaus, Marshall H., and Phyllis H. Klaus. *The Amazing Newborn*. Reading, Mass.: Addison-Wesley, 1985.

Konner, Melvin, "Symbolic Wound," *New York Times Magazine* (May 8, 1988):58.

Lagercrantz, Hugh, and Theodore A. Slotkin. "The 'Stress' of Being Born," *Scientific American* 254(Apr. 1986):100.

Leboyer, Frederick. *Birth Without Violence*. New York: Alfred A. Knopf, 1975.

Macfarlane, Aidan. *The Psychology of Childbirth*. Cambridge: Harvard University Press, 1977.

Maisels, M. Jeffrey. "Circumcision: The Effect of Information on Parental Decision Making," *Pediatrics* 71(1983):453.

Masciello, Anthony L. "Anesthesia for Neonatal Circumcision—Local Anesthesia is Better than Dorsal Penile Nerve Block," *Obstetrics and Gynecology* 75(1990):834.

Maxwell, Lynne G., et al. "Penile Nerve Block," *Obstetrics and Gynecology* 70(1987):415.

"Newborn Eye Treatments," *ICEA Review* 7:3(Dec. 1983).

Osborn, L.M., et al. "Hygienic Care in Uncircumcised Infants," *Pediatrics* 67(1981):365.

"Pediatricans Concede Circumcision Does Have Medical Benefits for Males," *Growing Child Research Review* 3(1989):4.

"Report of the Task Force on Circumcision," American Academy of Pediatrics Task Force on Circumcision, *Pediatrics* 84(1989):388.

Rothman, Barbara Katz. *Giving Birth.* New York: Penguin, 1984.

Schiff, Donald W. "American Academy of Pediatrics Member Alert," Mar. 10, 1989.

Weissbluth, Marc. *Crybabies.* New York: Berkeley, 1986.

Williamson, Paul S., and Marvel L. Williamson. "Physiologic Stress Reduction by a Local Anesthetic During Newborn Circumcision," *Pediatrics* 71(1983):36.

Wiswell, Thomas E., and Colonel Dietrich W. Geschke. "Risks from Circumcision During the First Month of Life Compared With Those for Uncircumcised Boys," *Pediatrics* 83(1989):10ll.

CHAPTER 20: EASING PAIN IN THE IMMEDIATE POSTPARTUM

Borovies, Dianne L. "Assessing and Managing Pain in Breast-Feeding Mothers," *MCN* 9(Jul.–Aug. 1984):272.

Brorup-Weston, Marianne, and Penny Simkin. "Cesarean Birth—A Special Delivery," available from Pennypress, Inc. (see Resources).

Cerutti, Edward R. "The Management of Breastfeeding," *Birth and the Family Journal* 8:4(1981):251.

deCarvalho, Manoel, et al. "Does the Duration and Frequency of Early Breastfeeding Affect Nipple Pain?" *Birth* 11:2(1984):81.

Dilts, Catherine L. "Nursing Management of Mastitis Due to Breastfeeding," *Journal of Obstetric, Gynecologic and Neonatal Nursing* 14(Jul.-Aug. 1985):286.

Droegemueller, William. "Cold Sitz Baths for Relief of Postpartum Perineal Pain," *Clinical Obstetrics and Gynecology* 23(Dec. 1980):1039.

Frink, Barbara, and Pamela Chally. "Managing Pain Responses to Cesarean Childbirth," *MCN* (Jul.–Aug. 1984):270.

Hollinger, Jan L. "Transcutaneous Electrical Nerve Stimulation After Cesarean Birth," *Physical Therapy* 66:1(1986):36.

Huggins, Kathleen. *The Nursing Mother's Companion,* revised edition. Boston: Harvard Common Press, 1991.

Leander, Kristine, and Jane Grassley. "Making Love After Birth," *Birth and the Family Journal* 7:3(1980):181.

L'Esperance, Carol, and Kittie Frantz. "Time Limitation for Early Breastfeeding," *Journal of Obstetric, Gynecologic and Neonatal Nursing* 14 (1985):114.

Lichtman, Ronnie, "Speedy Recovery," in *Childbirth '91.* Newton, Mass.: Cahners, 1991.

Lieberman, Adrienne, "Bosom Buddies," *American Baby* (January 1990):46.

Lim, Robin. *After the Baby's Birth . . . A Woman's Way to Wellness.* Berkeley: Celestial Arts, 1991.

Lozoff, Betsy. "Birth in Non-Industrial Societies," in *Birth, Interaction and Attachment,* M.H. Klaus and M.O. Robertson, eds. Skillman, New Jersey: Johnson and Johnson, 1982.

Rayburn, William F., et al. "Patient-Controlled Analgesia for Post-Cesarean Section Pain," *Obstetrics and Gynecology* 72(1988):136.

Riley, Judith E. "The Impact of Transcutaneous Electrical Nerve Stimulation on the Postcesarean Patient," *Journal of Obstetric, Gynecologic and Neonatal Nursing* 11(Sept.-Oct. 1982):325.

Woessner, Candace, et al. *Breastfeeding Today: A Mother's Companion.* Garden City Park, New York: Avery, 1987.

Wong, Shirley, and Elizabeth Stepp-Gilbert. "Lactation Suppression: Non-pharmaceutical versus Pharmaceutical Method," *Journal of Obstetric, Gynecologic and Neonatal Nursing* 14(Jul.–Aug. 1985):302.

INDEX